Shaping Childhood

Themes of uncertainty in the history of adult–child relationships

Roger Cox

Foreword by Olive Stevenson

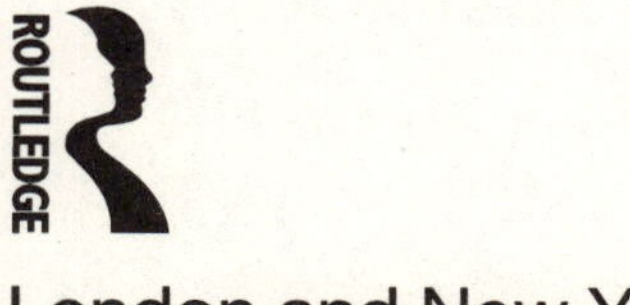

London and New York

First published 1996
by Routledge
11 New Fetter Lane, London EC4P 4EE

Simultaneously published in the USA and Canada
by Routledge
29 West 35th Street, New York, NY 10001

Typeset in Times by Routledge
Printed and bound in Great Britain by T. J. Press (Padstow) Ltd, Padstow, Cornwall

British Library Cataloguing in Publication Data
A catalogue record for this book is available from the British Library

Library of Congress Cataloguing in Publication Data
Cox, Roger, 1946–
Shaping childhood/themes of uncertainty in the history of adult–child relationships / Roger Cox : foreword by Olive Stevenson.
Includes bibliographical references and index. 1. Children – History. 2. Children and adults – History.
I. Title.
HQ767.87.C69 1997
305.23′09–dc20 96–7489

ISBN 0–415–11044–0

'But there wasn't a real dragon,' said the mother.

'It was just a story I made up.'

'It turned out to be true after all,' said the little boy.

'You should have looked in the match box first.'

'That is how it is,' said the lion. 'Some stories are true, and some aren't. . . . '

'A Lion in the Meadow' by Margaret Mahy

For my parents
and for
Maria

Contents

Foreword

As I read this book, images, sometimes unwelcome, crossed and recrossed my mind, testifying to the deep emotional significance of the topic and the power of the analysis. I remember, for example, my father's intense feelings as he sought to describe to his young daughter the concept of original sin. (It was part of a rationale for abandoning church.) His nostrils flared when emotions ran high and I see him now, positively twitching with distress at the idea of 'a little child being born sinful'. Born at the end of the nineteenth century, my father's feelings were still raw in the 1930s.

I remembered the tension surrounding the inquiry, in 1973, into the death of Maria Colwell at the hands of her stepfather. I was a member of the inquiry and I argued with my colleagues. In particular, I recall an acrimonious exchange as to whether it was culturally acceptable for a 6-year-old child, in a council housing estate in the early 1970s, to collect bags of coal from the shop, in a pram, for her mother.

I remember the shock, when, a year or two ago, someone gave me a book of Charles Dodgson's photographs of pubescent girls. The revulsion which I felt was quite visceral. The photographs are no longer in my house. They formed the core of a short story on sexual abuse which I attempted at a 'creative writing course' last year.

These three examples illustrate some of the dimensions of the subject of childhood which are significant: social influences, filtered by parents; sociological awareness and powerful subjective reactions to sexuality, shaped by contemporary values.

I am not an expert in the history of childhood but I have been, for some forty years, continuously involved, professionally and academically, with child welfare, particularly those aspects concerned with the protection of children against abuse. Since the 1970s there has been mounting public interest in the issue; the media has raised public indignation, both at the failure of the authorities (notably social workers) to protect children and at their unwarrantable intrusion into family life. The complexity of the subject has spawned a huge professional and academic literature and fostered an international network of 'experts' in the field. Certain phrases to describe abuse ('a social construct') or its consequences ('a moral panic') or associated concepts ('cultural relativism') have become clichés in the discourse. As the years have gone by, and much influenced by the US, particular dimensions have been emphasised. Thus, in the 1970s, the debate was largely concentrated on 'non accidental injury'; in the 1980s, the searchlight turned on sexual abuse. Not surprisingly, this has proved powerfully contentious, particularly when it has been linked to suggestions of ritualistic and 'Satanic' connections. Such allegations took the subject into the religious arena, with counter allegations that fundamentalist Christians wished to find Evil (however slim the evidence) so that they could banish it with Good. The ripples went wider; in the US, the fundamentalist 'tendency' was linked to right-wing politics. It is easy to see in this the making of myth which expresses deep dilemmas and tensions in society. However, disturbingly, in a welter of accusation and counter accusation, there can be no doubt that organised abusers, such as those in paedophiliac rings, have played a sinister part in creating a climate in which fearful things happen to children.

In the face of such intense and alarming phenomena, it becomes very important for academics and professionals concerned with contemporary social policy and intervention to have a sense of historical context about childhood, to understand something of the origins of our present confusions. Unfortunately, such historical awareness has not been a feature of current literature, most of which at best surveys the history of child abuse in a superficial and selective way.

One theme, in particular, stands out for me and is beautifully illustrated in these pages. Put quite baldly, it concerns the 'natural' goodness or badness of children. Would my father's abhorrence of the concept of original sin have been shaken by the Bulger case? Or would he by now have been influenced by the discourse which stresses the effects of familial and environmental deficits on the developing child? In the 1970s, we sought in child welfare policy to abandon the distinction between the 'deprived' and the 'depraved' child. In the 1980s, with a very proper concern that children alleging sexual abuse had not been listened to, some professionals absurdly argued that children 'always told the truth'. More seriously, however, there was the question – if they do not always tell the truth is it because they are afraid, ambivalent or muddled? Or are they just plain naughty? In the 1990s, in the public utterances of politicians, these distinctions have been reinstated; children are either 'villains' or 'victims'. They cannot be both.

Psychoanalytic theories, especially those of Melanie Klein and Donald Winnicott, offer a perspective on this seeming inability to integrate notions of goodness and badness. Many hundreds of pages are devoted to the phenomenon of 'splitting' the emotions of love and hate and of the psychic task of integration. Even this, however, as this book shows, is founded on a relatively recent concept of a developmental process called childhood.

This book offers an important analysis, spanning several hundred years and richly illustrated, of the relationships between adults and children or, rather, what the adults said about them and about the nature of children. Those of us who struggle with the here and now have, I think, a moral duty (as well as an intellectual impetus) to seek to understand better the powerful emotions and confused thoughts which beset us when we need to take action about children. As this book shows so well, these emotions and thoughts are rooted in our corporate and individual history.

Olive Stevenson
Emeritus Professor of Social Work Studies
University of Nottingham

Acknowledgements

I would like first to remember Jean Heywood, the first Children's Officer of the small Lancashire borough of Rochdale and later a lecturer at the University of Manchester, whose interest in the history of childhood first awakened my own and who could always find relevance in sources from well beyond her own specialised field. Her view of the child was one of the most 'interdisciplinary' that I have yet come across. I should also like to thank the generations of students who have long-sufferingly allowed me to inflict on them material which they never thought was part of the deal they signed up for. It is greatly to their credit that the 'Childhood and Society' course has survived for so many years. More specifically, I should like to thank the School of Social Studies for allowing me the time to collect my ideas together into some manageable form, and the librarians of the Briggs Special Collection of Educational Literature in the Hallward Library of Nottingham University, not only for finding books even when the old cataloguing system (soon to be computerised) failed them, but also for providing a place of refuge when inspiration failed. I am particularly grateful to Professor Olive Stevenson who has agreed to introduce this study to its readers for me. She, like many of my colleagues in the School, has been remarkably tolerant of my inability to engage directly with contemporary policy. This study is by way of a small peace offering.

The author and publisher would like to thank the following for the use of copyright material: HarperCollins Publishers for Rousseau's *Emile, or On Education*, 1979, translated by Allan Bloom; Oxford University Press for Locke's *Some Thoughts Concerning Education*, 1989, edited by J. W. and J. S. Yolton; J. M. Dent for *The Lion in the Meadow*, 1969, by Margaret Mahy.

Chapter 1

The child in history

Introduction

The history of childhood does not have a particularly auspicious past. It is itself an illustration of a process which is one of the themes of this book; namely the process whereby an idea takes flight, and having been let loose upon the world it reaches unexpected places, acquires unexpected meanings and becomes the subject of controversy, a pawn in battles that occasionally have little to do with its origins. Any account of this history, however brief, must start with Ariès' *Centuries of Childhood*, the original French edition of which was published in 1960 and was translated into English by 1962 (Ariès, 1973). Moving from his earlier studies of demographic history to the realm of culture, and drawing on evidence relating to paintings of children, to their clothes, their games and their schooling as well as to their representation in family iconography, Ariès explored the origins of the originality of the modern nuclear family. But the idea that caught the popular imagination, the great discovery that Ariès appeared to have launched upon the world, was that in pre-modern times there was no conception of childhood and that consequently childhood must be regarded as the product of modern western societies. In an often quoted passage Ariès said:

> In medieval society the idea of childhood did not exist; this is not to suggest that children were neglected, forsaken or despised. The idea of childhood is not to be confused with affection for children; it corresponds to an awareness of the particular nature of childhood, that particular nature which distinguishes the child from the adult, even the young adult. In medieval society, this awareness was lacking. That is why, as soon as the child could live without the constant solicitude of his mother, his nanny or his cradle-rocker, he belonged to adult society. That adult society now strikes us as

> rather puerile: no doubt this is largely a matter of its mental age, but it is also due to its physical age, because it was partly made up of children and youths.
>
> (Ariès, 1973: 125)

In spite of Ariès' careful distinction here between a mental concept and everyday behaviour, the book was widely interpreted as saying that nobody could have experienced being a child until the idea of childhood had been invented. As Vann notes, the history of this idea (for in the minds of most this *was* the book) reads like a picaresque novel (Vann, 1982). Outside the field of history, especially within the teaching of social sciences to undergraduates and within the training of professionals whose work related to childhood, the Ariès 'idea' rapidly gained hold. On the one hand it encouraged a belief in human progress; no matter that Ariès thought the high point for the child was in the seventeenth century, back home from medieval apprenticeship and service but not yet sent to modern school! On the other hand, its implicit cultural relativism opened up the possibility of more liberal interpretations of the possibilities of childhood. Children might gain rights of their own and perhaps share in women's escape from the oppression of patriarchal society. In a sense the Ariès idea seemed to offer the best of all worlds. We now, at least, had a concept of childhood, so we would not ill-treat children or fail to respect their special needs, as presumably happened before childhood was invented. But we could also throw off the shackles of contemporary practices, especially those which constrained the child within an overly protective and restrictive schedule, since these had no foundation except in history.

Historians for their part were, on the whole, always less than enraptured, not least because Ariès was seen as an interloper into a field he did not really understand (Wilson, 1980). This feeling was intensified, perhaps, by the concurrent enthusiasm for psychological interpretations of history which, whilst they produced some insightful studies of parenting and childhood in the past, also spawned grand theory in a manner antithetical to many professional historians (Hunt, 1972; Demos, 1970). For example, Lloyd de Mause's psychogenic interpretation of the history of childhood, in which adults through the course of history grow ever more in empathy with their offspring, had none of the sophistication of Ariès and employed all manner of evidence as proof of actual behaviour (de Mause, 1976). To this was joined the elegant social history of Lawrence Stone who, with infinitely more command of history, sketched a transformation amongst upper-class families in the seventeenth and eighteenth centuries especially, which placed the changing nature of the parent–child relationship at its heart. To the idea of the history of childhood he contributed the notion of 'affective individualism' in the family, a growing ideal amongst parents committed not only to each other, but also to raising their children through love and respect (Stone, 1979). Whilst Stone recognised a growing variety in human conduct, he too seemed incautiously to interpret behaviour directly from sources of evidence that spoke much more of governing ideas than actual practices (Pollock, 1983). There were other objections, too, to Stone's interpretations. To some, his was a narrative too accepting of orthodox sociological modernisation theories in which 'individualism' rises with capitalism to dominate the *mentalité* of all western societies (Macfarlane, 1979); others were simply wary of the scope and all-inclusive nature of the interpretation (Houlbrooke, 1984).

But perhaps the most important challenge to the idea initiated by Ariès, and given impetus by de Mause and Stone, came from those historians who were unwilling to accept that so basic a human state as childhood could be subject to the whim of historical change. This reversal of approach threatened to deny the possibility of serious change in the state of childhood at all. At its best in the work of historians like Pollock, it produced a sober and realistic interpretation of the experience of childhood in the past (Pollock, 1983). But Pollock was wary of abandoning the possibility of historical change in relation to childhood and warned against too abrupt a 'volte-face in the historiography of family life'. Urging the need 'to cultivate a sense of proportion in our contemporary interpretation of change', she argued that,

> Change and continuity should be investigated simultaneously, the one concept informing the other. Instead of searching for the existence or absence of emotions such as love, grief, or anger, we should concede that these emotions will be present in all cultures and in all communities, and seek instead for the varied ways in which they were perceived and expressed in particular societies.
>
> (Pollock, 1987: 12)

The problem lay as much as anywhere in the evidence that was available. Access to historical material which tells us much about the experience of childhood is all too rare. Much has to be inferred from sources which are 'idealistic' rather than descriptive; domestic conduct books, literary sources, travellers' tales, writing designed to instruct or entertain the young themselves. The problem is that, not only does such material leave open the question whether real experience can be implied from it, but it often has another ideological agenda of its own. The consequence of this is that interpretation is drawn away from experience towards these other agendas within the terms of which experience is then explained. It is this process which leads historians like Stone to elaborate explanations of experience in terms of theories which encompass the development of western societies as a whole. An ambitious sociologist, armed with systematically collected evidence including the subject's own interpretation, might attempt such explanations of contemporary experience, but rarely is such material left us by history.

The shift Pollock implies, away from investigating experience towards an examination of 'perceptions' and 'expression', is therefore significant. Though Pollock's own study of childhood experience through an examination of diaries and autobiographies remains one of the most important of its kind, she herself found conclusions difficult to draw, precisely because lived experience is so various, so contingent and so unclear. In fact, Ariès himself was well aware of this, emphasising that his study was of the 'idea' of the family, not of the everyday experience of living within a family (Ariès, 1973: 8, 393). More recently there has been a re-emphasis of important themes in his work; of his account of a growing perception of linear time with its enormous implications for conceptions of the life-cycle, and of the growth of the notion of discipline especially within the emerging institution of the school (Hutton, 1981; Casey, 1989). Hunt, like Hutton, believes that Ariès should be understood alongside scholars like Elias and Foucault, as one who studied 'long range trends in the alteration of the structure of the psyche' (Hunt, 1986: 217). What Ariès identified, according to Hutton, was the 'gathering complexity' of the mental structures which accumulate through the civilising process, and in so doing he explored 'the paradox that such mental structures are at once the essential mode of human creativity and the primary obstacle to it' (Hutton, 1981: 242).

In the wider field, too, beyond the narrower boundaries of history, there was a change in the nature of references to Ariès' work. As the clouds of pessimism gathered in the late 1980s and 1990s, it was increasingly accepted that there was an historical legacy that needed to be better understood, and that our own dealings with children were shaped by past conceptions that would not easily go away (Hendrick,

1990; Stainton Rogers, 1992; Best, 1994). There was a growing appreciation too, that though the historical perspective offered a successive variety of childhoods, at any one time one version was seeking dominance. As Hendrick puts it, 'each construction sought to speak of "childhood" as a singular noun; the plural posed too many conceptual and political problems' (Hendrick, 1990: 55).

There is a sense in which the legacy of Ariès, though by different routes through the realms of social science and history, has lead to similar conclusions. These briefly stated are simple enough. First that childhood is a socially constructed concept which varies by time, geography, culture, and economic and social status. Second that the relationship between the biological child and the social construction of childhood is complex and produces the varied lived experiences of children, difficult to assess in the present, frequently deeply inaccessible in the past. And third, that we can attempt to understand our current preoccupations, ambiguities and anxieties about childhood by seeing them as part of a legacy from the past, a past which seems to exert a hold upon us whether or not we would wish to be free of it.

Methodologically, too, it seems that the approach to the history of childhood adopted by Ariès still appears to offer fruitful opportunities. It took another marginal historian however, Michel Foucault, to provide the framework. His is a complex and controversial legacy which cannot be fully discussed here, but the coupling of his name by historians like Hunt and Hutton to that of Ariès suggests important possibilities. Foucault does not offer a systematic theory after the manner of Marx or Freud, nor a tightly organised methodology (Sheridan, 1980: 225). Rather what he does offer is room for manoeuvre, the space to offer limited accounts in a field which has been bedeviled by the influence of grand narrative. In the first place, Foucault like Ariès was prepared to spend his time in the study of traditionally insignificant groups. He turned his attention to deviants of all kinds and claimed for them a significance in the cultural and institutional formations of modern societies. In the same way, Ariès had first suggested that the insignificant child stood at the centre of a major alteration in the way the life-cycle was perceived in western society. Foucault also attempted to redefine power and to move attention away from the centre (the state, social and economic elites) to the periphery. He wished it to be seen, not as originating in and flowing from politics or economics, nor as something 'possessed' by the powerful, but rather as 'an infinitely complex network of "micro-powers", of power relations that permeate every aspect of social life' (Sheridan, 1980: 139; O'Brien, 1989). Perhaps most importantly, Foucault saw power not simply as an exercise in repressive control, but as something that could also be driven by the need to be productive and creative. There are problems with any theory of power that appears to deny the enduring structures power creates, but at least in relation to childhood, Foucault's conception serves to remind us that even the earliest and most intimate relations between child and adult are, in some sense, relations of power.

Perhaps most of all, Foucault developed the rather loose and baggy, but always useful concept of a discourse. At its simplest, a discourse is a social process in which, through language (used in its broadest sense to include all semiotic systems) we make sense of the world around us, but also the process by which the world makes sense of us (O'Sullivan et al., 1994). Discourses, thus, construct society by constructing 'objects of knowledge, social subjects and forms of "self", social relationships and conceptual frameworks' (Fairclough, 1992: 39). A particular discursive formation will construct objects and relationships according to a particular set of rules which help to formulate 'technologies of power', and clearly some will be more successful than others. As children we are born into something which resembles a primordial soup of discourses; these represent the world to us and at the same time position us as individuals within that world (Hodge and Kress, 1988: 240). Access to discourses can be sought through the examination of texts which can be thought of as containing elements of discourse. Here a text is no more than any convenient assemblage of signs, indicative of the meanings we attribute to some aspect of human life. In practical terms, they may be stories, poems, letters, diaries, conversations, domestic conduct books, sermons, pictures and photographs, ways of dressing, ways of eating, ways of making love – anything which packages the cultural meaning of everyday life into a form that can be examined. They are one important means by which the knowledge that discourses create is codified, circulated and reinforced. They can also be the means by which discourses are challenged and rejected. Texts should never be taken as straightforward accounts of discourse; reading them is an act of interpretation. A text, as Hodge and Kress note, is 'only a trace of discourses, frozen and preserved, more or less reliable or misleading' (1988: 12).

It is possible to re-read Ariès as a study of the emergence of various discourses relating to childhood, in particular the developmental discourse with all its ramifications for the entry of the child into adult life, and the discourse of discipline within which the child was located as a creature over whom power was to be exercised productively. His texts are the paintings, the games, the clothes of the first part of his book and the educational tracts and orders for the running of schools which make up much of the second part. Such a reading is not unproblematic, but it does serve to re-establish the important agenda which Ariès set. It will not solve the problem of understanding the actual experience of children, but it defines more clearly how close and how far we are from that experience. From the traces in the text to the discourse and on to the experience is a long journey, but at least in attempting to understand the discourse we are attempting to understand a structure of meaning to which experience has, of necessity, to relate.

Discourses come and go. They can vary from the short-lived, localised and explicitly articulated (the early historiography of childhood discussed above would be an example) to much more deep-seated ways of understanding the world (religious beliefs, for example). When dominant, these latter, because they are so embedded in culture, become naturalised and, though constantly elaborated upon, their basic propositions are assumed rather than expressly articulated. To take one example, the assumption of a gradual, linear development from infancy to adulthood is now so accepted that we rarely question it. Such discourses may only come under public scrutiny when some event suddenly challenges their presuppositions, as for example when, after a brief holiday romance, a 13-year-old English girl leaves home with her parents' blessing to marry an 18-year-old Turkish waiter and live in a remote Turkish town. The reason we find the age of 13 too young is because we accept, largely without question, the strictures of a range of influential discourses which define a 13-year-old girl as a child, socially and sexually immature. Discourses can achieve great significance but rarely complete dominance. Many are always in competition, always explicitly intertextual in the sense that their articulation depends upon opposition to or support for other pre-existing texts pertaining to other discourses. The concepts generated through these discourses live on to enter other discourses often with altered meanings, and especially with significantly different emotive and cognitive connotations. In some cases, there is a constant reference back to history, indeed a constant rewriting of history in order to reshape a particular concept in the light of the needs of current discourse. Foucault preferred to talk of 'beginnings' rather than 'origins' and of 'genealogies' rather than 'causes', because the history of any discourse has many possible beginnings and much wasted energy can be spent in deciding where the real origins are. The interest lies rather in exploring differences and in finding the disturbances that threaten any orthodoxy.

The historical part of this book is largely concerned with these intertextualities, with the way in which concepts generated by particular discourses both depend upon earlier concepts which they use or abuse to their own ends and at the same time contribute to later discourses. Roughly speaking, there are two types of discourses examined here. Two of them, those relating to Puritanism and to Romanticism, have fairly specific historic origins. These, although they have genealogies traceable to a remote past, also have identifiable beginnings represented by clear differences from their surrounding discourses. The other two, dealing with the Enlightenment and with Victorian discourses on gender and sexuality in childhood, are slightly different. Although they are specifically located historically (and in the case of the Enlightenment, very narrowly located textually in the work of Locke and Rousseau), they do deal with more existential questions – with the rationality and sexuality of the child. However, the distinction should not be drawn too sharply; the question of original sin, though it is posed in an historically specific way by the Puritans, raises existential questions about the moral nature of the child, and, however basic questions relating to the child's sexuality seem to be, their enunciation in the late nineteenth century is historically very specific.

In the rest of this study an attempt has been made to try and ensure that the somewhat abstract theoretical language employed in this discussion does not obtrude too much. Demonstrations of academic virility are all very well in their way, but they can make the analysis feel unnecessarily cumbersome and be alienating to the non-specialist reader. There are occasions when it is inevitable that some specialist language is employed, especially when a particular writer offers a strongly theoretical interpretation (Anthony Easthope on Wordsworth is a clear example). These occasional excursions into a more rarefied language have been introduced in the belief that something of particular significance is offered by the writers concerned. Readers are invited to give them due attention, but in the end must make their own judgement. In a short study of this kind, there is a very heavy reliance upon secondary sources and this, to some degree, determines also the kind of evidence that has been employed. Different discourses have their origins in different places, and this is reflected in the kind of secondary sources used. Puritanism was born of a religious and political movement, the Enlightenment was essentially an intellectual enterprise, and Romanticism was primarily a literary movement; as a consequence secondary sources range from social history to intellectual history and literary criticism. It is one of the pleasures of engaging in a study of this kind to note the increasing interdisciplinarity of much modern scholarship. One source of primary evidence has, however, been used in several different contexts; this is writing designed specifically for children, mostly in the form of poetry or stories. Whilst there is a well developed specialist field of study in children's literature, it has perhaps been under-used in more general discussions of the history of childhood. Yet it is a source that deserves more extensive and detailed examination than it can receive here, since through writing directly to children, authors (often conscious of their multiple roles as writers, educators and even parents) most clearly express their own hopes, fears and expectations for and of the children of the rising generation.

There are also notable absences from this study. The child at school has been marginalised as has the child who falls under the shadow of the state in other ways. There is little reference to the impact of science even though it could claim to have shaped much nineteenth- and twentieth-century discourse about the child. It would have been possible, too, and entirely appropriate to say much more about the mother–child dyad. There are various justifications that could be offered for their omission. They are all discourses with such strong intertextualities (in schooling and the curriculum; in politics; within the important scientific disciplines of medicine and psychology themselves; within feminist studies) that it would have been all too easy for the focus to slip away from the child into other areas. It is also true that each of these fields has its own extensive and important literature which makes demands upon discussion and analysis that a short text cannot easily deal with. But at the end of the day, the selection is personal and eclectic, reflecting an individual history of exploration. It is, in fact, easy to get trapped by others' orthodoxies; to ignore the Puritans because they largely pre-date the great intellectual endeavours of the Enlightenment; to get caught by the increasingly self-reverential musings of developmental psychology as the old certainties about socialisation slip away; to allow the ungendered child to fall into a void created by an over-insistence upon gendered analysis. The selection here may inadequately

Chapter 2

The child of Puritanism

The making of an historical myth

> Come, my Children, let us pack up and be gone to the Gate that leads to the Celestial Country, that we may see your Father, and be with him and his Companions in peace, according to the Laws of that Land.
>
> Then did her Children burst out into tears of joy that the heart of their Mother was so inclined.
>
> John Bunyan,
> *The Pilgrim's Progress: The Second Part*

Many problems confront twentieth-century students of Puritanism, but two in particular are likely to be most persistent. One has to do with the inescapable fact that Puritanism must be understood as the product of religious belief. And as Margarita Stocker says, 'religion in a period as proud of its scepticism as our own evokes and offends all manner of prejudices' (Stocker, 1992: 53). If we are not to be glib or even flippant in our judgement of Puritan child-rearing aims and practices, we need to feel the depth of belief in heaven and hell, in the sinfulness of human beings and in the boundless grace of God that could be felt by a Puritan parent, and to acknowledge as real the anguish as well as the joy that such belief might bring to the parents of a growing child.

The other major problem is that Puritanism does not come to us directly across the intervening centuries, but is shaped by the evaluations, perceptions and prejudices of many who have lived in between; we look back at the Puritans through a lens not of our own making. Thus, writing of seventeenth-century Massachusetts, the most important of the Puritan colonies of New England, Edmund Morgan says it has become to the modern mind 'a preposterous land of witches and witch hunters, kill-joys in tall-crowned hats, whose main occupation was to prevent each other from having any fun and whose sole virtue lay in their furniture' (Morgan, 1958: xi). Lawrence

Sasek, too, has noted how American descendants of the New England settlers will open 'Puritan' restaurants and hotels, use the word as a product label and even proudly boast their Puritan origins, but would be most offended to be called Puritan themselves (Sasek, 1989: 2). Because Puritans offend our moral complacency, Morgan suggests, we caricature them in order to feel comfortable in their presence. Late twentieth-century liberal, professional communities pride themselves upon their tolerance and cultural awareness, but not infrequently use historical myths of past incompetence or supposed ignorance to highlight their own superior knowledge. Perhaps nowhere is this more evident than in the use of the term Puritan as a term of abuse when applied to parenting.

Anyone seeking to gain an understanding of the impact of Puritanism upon the cultural history of childhood has to confront two conflicting accounts of its effect upon the perception of childhood, and upon parental approaches to the business of child-rearing. The first account is critical, seeing Puritanism as the enemy of all that is progressive, reasonable and loving. The second sees Puritans as the pioneers of the bourgeois family, the advocates of a rational, ordered and serious approach to the business of social reproduction. Puritans, it is held, transferred the discipline of incipient capitalism to the domestic scene and framed it within a religion that was rescued from the remote church and established round the hearth. This chapter will attempt to unpick these apparently contradictory accounts, to show how our contemporary understanding has and still is being shaped.

One thing, however, is clear; the preoccupations of Puritan parents have, in late twentieth-century folk wisdom, been unduly trivialised, as has the meaning of Puritanism itself. If one of the simpler uses of historical understanding is to challenge our contemporary perceptions, an exploration of the fate of the Puritan movement is not merely a search to understand something remote from our everyday concerns – an act of duty – but also a search to understand and perhaps challenge the basis of our own rejection of what we believe Puritanism stands for.

THE REPRESSIVE PURITAN

The first and most 'popular' story about Puritanism presents an image of exclusiveness and bigotry and of children being raised in a repressive and claustrophobic environment, living narrow, rigid lives dominated by religious observance. Puritanism could certainly be used as a term of abuse in the late sixteenth century (Hill, 1964: 13), but there is little indication that when it was so used it was directed against the methods of child-rearing Puritans employed. As with many of our most powerful images of the past, the image of the repressive Puritan parent comes to us through subsequent representations which have acquired a life of their own. Twentieth-century arrogance is particularly critical of the narrow 'Puritanism' of the Victorian age, but much of that criticism is itself based upon nineteenth-century critiques of Puritanism and its heirs.

The popular image of Puritanism is easy to identify and to maintain. There are examples of Puritan preachers, such as John Robinson in 1628, thundering out the sinfulness of youth:

> And surely, there is in all children, though not alike, a stubbornness, and stoutness of mind arising from natural pride, which must, in the first place, be broken and beaten down. . . . This fruit of natural corruption and root of actual rebellion both against God and man must be destroyed.
>
> (quoted Stannard, 1977: 49)

Or the New England preacher Cotton Mather in 1689:

> They go astray as soon as they are born. They no sooner *step* than they *stray*, they no sooner *lisp* than they *ly*. Satan gets them to be proud, profane, reviling and revengeful as *young* as they are.
>
> (quoted Stannard, 1977: 50)

Then there is James Janeway's *A Token for Children: Being An Exact Account of the Conversion, Holy and Exemplary Lives and Joyful Deaths of Several Young Children*, published in 1671, in the preface of which he confronts his child readers with the consequences of sin:

> And are you willing to go to hell to be burned with the devil and his angels? Would you be in the same condition as naughty children? Oh, hell is a terrible place, that is worse a thousand times than whipping; God's anger is worse than your father's anger! and are you willing to anger God? O child, this is most certainly true, that all that be wicked, and die so, must be turned into hell; and if any be once there, there is no coming out again.

And, of course there is always Susanna Wesley, mother of John, the founder of methodism, who in 1732 advised her son that she had taught all her children to 'fear the rod and to cry softly', adding somewhat chillingly 'by which means they escaped abundance of correction which they might otherwise have had' (quoted Tomalin, 1981: 14).

What is less often said, however, is that Robinson, though he may have been the original 'Pilgrim Pastor', wrote and offered his advice as a voluntary exile in Holland and that those whom he inspired set up the separatist colony of Plymouth. If there is such a thing as a mainstream Puritan, the description could probably not be applied to John Robinson. Equally, whilst Cotton Mather was of a more mainstream New England background, he was of the third generation and, as we shall see later in this chapter, several writers believe there was a dynamic in Puritanism that rendered later generations much more anxious about the salvation of their children than their grandparents had been.

As far as Janeway is concerned, what kept his book alive was not the preface but the stories themselves, which, though they read strangely to the twentieth-century mind, were engaging and persuasive enough to fascinate that arch rationalist William Godwin as a child. He must have read the book in the 1760s and later recalled that it inspired him to try to achieve something great in his own life. Cotton Mather, incidentally, attempted something similar to Janeway but clearly lacked the same literary skill (Sommerville, 1992: 57). And as for Susanna Wesley's so often quoted remark, it is well worth putting it back into the homely context where it belongs, bearing in mind that, having given birth to nineteen children, ten of whom survived infancy, Susanna presided over a large and potentially unruly household:

> The children were always put into a regular method of living, in such things as they were capable of, from their birth; as in dressing and undressing, changing their linen etc. The first quarter commonly passed in sleep. After that they were, if possible, laid into their cradle awake, and rocked to sleep, and so they were kept rocking until it was time for them to awake. This was done to bring them to a regular course of sleeping, which at first was three hours in the morning, and three in the afternoon; afterwards two hours, till they needed none at all. When they turned a year old (and some before) they were taught to fear the rod and to cry softly, by which means they escaped abundance of correction which they might otherwise have had, and that most odious noise of crying of children was rarely heard in the house, but the family

usually lived in as much quietness as if there had not been a child among them.

(quoted in Tomalin, 1981: 14)

Mrs Wesley seems more to deserve our admiration for her household management skills than opprobrium as one of the folk-devils of oppressively religious parenting.

None of this, of course, is to deny that Puritans and their dissenting and evangelical heirs viewed children as sinners with distressingly unsaintly habits; and that, as sinners, children were in need of salvation and, as human beings, in need of good manners. But we know so little about the actual lives of these people that it ill-behoves us to extrapolate everyday behaviour from the utterances of preachers. For they were caught up in a movement that had far greater ambitions than could conceivably be encompassed by child-rearing. Nor should we judge on the basis of a collection of stories whose power now so completely eludes us, or from mere phrases snatched from their context.

THE TAYLORS OF ONGAR

The problem of how to approach the parenting of the original Puritans will be considered in more detail later in this chapter, but for the moment it is worth trying to counter the myth of the repressed Puritan family with an example of just one dissenting family who lived and worked around the end of the eighteenth and the beginning of the nineteenth centuries. Certainly social historians have found plenty of evidence of 'Puritan' attitudes and behaviour at this time. Davidoff and Hall (1987), for example, find many echoes of seventeenth-century Puritan doctrines in the evangelical revivals, and see these as significant in the development of nineteenth-century middle-class family life.

The Taylors of Ongar as they came to be known provide an interesting example. Accounts of the lives of Ann and Jane Taylor and their siblings, and of their parents, Isaac and Ann, describe a family that experienced its fair share of economic insecurity, illness and death, and even a certain amount of persecution and social isolation before reaching a degree of stability and, through their literary endeavours, even distinction (Armitage, 1939; Stewart, 1975; Davidoff and Hall, 1987). It is a story of a family whose 'defence and sense of place came through their religion and their family' (Davidoff and

Hall, 1987: 68). The way Isaac and Ann Taylor sought to bring up their children, and strove to integrate living, working, learning and religious observance within the household, says much for the influence of the old Puritan desire for the 'spiritualisation of the household'. Isaac, in particular, is reported as rising early and praying for an hour each morning in his closet, often aloud so that the children were aware of how emotional an experience it was.

But the education was far from being a narrow religious one. Ann Taylor, the mother, recalled that at breakfast time for many years she read to her husband, primarily to keep her own mind active, but the growing children also became used to listening and Mrs Taylor commented upon 'the incalculable benefit arising to the children of the family from the volumes they have thus heard read.... It is scarcely conceivable at what an early age they thus obtained gleanings of knowledge' (quoted in Armitage, 1939: 9). Ann and Jane were taught engraving, the family business, and also learned the skills of household management, wifehood and motherhood through their mother, though Jane never married and died of cancer at the age of 41. As little girls they were required to look after themselves and, according to Armitage, had 'a small room . . . allotted to them' where they 'dressed their dolls, whipped their tops and lived in a fairy land of the imagination' (Armitage, 1939: 14). Sketches of their earliest poems were found in the margins of plans of fortified towns which their father had given them to label with the correct names of 'fosses', 'bastions', and so on.

Discipline, one suspects, was not so different from that which obtained in the Wesley household. Ann, in her autobiography, makes reference to the fact that her parents became known as 'good managers' of children who refused to 'suffer *humoured* children to disturb either themselves or their friends'. She wrote,

> There is scarcely an expression so fraught to my earliest recollection with ideas of disgrace and misery as that of the 'humoured child', and I should have felt truly ashamed to exhibit one of my own at my father's table.
>
> (quoted in Darton, 1982: 184)

She herself was, according to a family friend, equally firm with her own children. She taught them,

> at one year old to sit quite still on her knee during family worship, and to understand that the toy or biscuit which might be in the

> hand must be laid aside till the conclusion of the service; and this was universally done without murmur.
>
> (Armitage, 1939: 107)

As a grandmother, she clearly had not lost her touch:

> Yesterday, before he [Ann's grandson] was brought as usual to my room, he indulged in a long continued violent thoroughly *manufactured* scream. Hitherto I have greeted his arrival with truly grandmotherly demonstrations of love and joy, but on this occasion I felt it wise to wear the calm appearance of deep silent sorrow, not bestowing a word or a smile.
>
> (Armitage, 1939: 107)

Grandson apparently understood. Such a family serves to connect the Puritan tradition of the seventeenth century to the twentieth century. In their everyday concerns about and behaviour towards children, they are not so unfamiliar to us; nor would they have been to their Puritan forbears. Their solidarity and cohesiveness remain attractive and they demonstrate clearly how a deep and emotional seriousness about the business of child-rearing and education can also be creative and pleasurable. Isaac and Ann manifested not only a concern for children, but a willingness to invest resources of both time and emotional energy, and they saw religion as a source of joy not fear (Davidoff and Hall, 1987: 63). When, in due course, the family began to break up, they agreed at Isaac's instigation, every full moon, to pause at nine in the evening, look at the moon and think of each other.

But at the level of their literary work, the fate of Ann and Jane Taylor's poetry illustrates the tensions and the contradictions of the nineteenth century and its attitude to the Puritan tradition. Their parents were born in the mid-eighteenth century, both from dissenting backgrounds, religion being, according to Davidoff and Hall, the principal legacy which Isaac was left by his father. According to family legend they also inherited something more tangible since Isaac possessed a copy of Dr Isaac Watts' *Divine Songs Attempted in Easy Language for the Use of Children*. First published in 1715, this family heirloom had been given to Isaac's grandmother by the author himself when, as a little girl, she sat on his knee. This book itself could stand as a symbol for the growth and decline of Puritan influence on child-rearing. Darton claims that Watts represented the 'end of the Puritan aggressive, persecuting, frightened love of children', which is probably a calumny against his predecessors (Darton, 1982: 108; Sommerville, 1992). But that aside, for more than a hundred years Watts' book was one of the principal tools in the articulation of the relationship between adult and child. However, by the time Lewis Carroll came to write his *Alice* books in the 1860s, Watts' songs had become the subject of parody. The 'little busy bee' who sought to improve each shining hour had become Carroll's 'little crocodile' with a narcissistic interest in its tail, and the voice of the sluggard had been metamorphosed into that of Carroll's lobster.

But Watts' legacy was also more specific. As Darton notes, the verse that Watts wrote for children was unrivalled until Ann and Jane themselves began to write for children early in the nineteenth century (Darton, 1982: 110). Their concern was certainly moral, but so is that of most contemporary children's poetry, and in their *Hymns for Infant Minds*, published in 1810, they wrote in the preface that they aimed to adopt 'evangelical truths to the wants and feelings of childhood in a language which it understands'. Modern commentators are generally impressed by the content and by the craft which the young women employed in consciously attempting to follow in Isaac Watts' footsteps, and certainly there is in their poetry a perception of the real world of children, its incidents and preoccupations.

Unfortunately, their poetry is now mostly known only through parodies. Jane, author of *Twinkle, Twinkle Little Star*, suffered, like Watts, at the hands of Carroll – the twinkling star, it may be recalled, was turned unceremoniously into a twinkling bat – and both provided models for Belloc in his *Cautionary Tales* (Darton, 1982: 111; Hunt, 1994; Grylls, 1978). Didactic both Watts and the Taylors undoubtedly were, and by no means averse to employing threats. Harry, for example, in Jane Taylor's *The Little Fisherman*, is rewarded for taking pleasure in fishing by catching his chin on a large meat hook from which he dangles,

> While from his wounds the crimson blood
> In dreadful torrents poured.

Sentimental they could also be after the manner of Watts' portrait of the infant Jesus in his *Cradle Hymn*, the popularity of which survived well into the twentieth century. Perhaps Ann's most famous poem was 'My Mother', which begins,

> Who fed me from her gentle breast,

And hush'd me in her arms to rest,
And on my cheek sweet kisses 'prest?
My Mother.

When sleep forsook my open eye,
Who was it sung sweet hushabye,
And rocked me that I should not cry?
My Mother.

Such verse lends itself to parody and 'My Mother' certainly achieved recognition through parody throughout the nineteenth century. Bertrand Russell certainly knew an indelicate school-boy version, and it perhaps received its last such memorial with Terry Scott's rendering of 'My Brother' well into the second half of the twentieth century. The business of parody itself is testimony not only to the popularity of verse such as this, but also to the fact that it was not treated with quite the reverence which we sometimes attribute to the nineteenth-century attitudes to childhood and motherhood.

The history of 'My Mother' presents us with another intriguing glimpse of the changing attitudes towards religion and to the way in which religion should be employed in child-rearing. The original last verse is as follows:

For God who lives above the skies,
Would look with vengeance in His eyes,
If I should ever dare despise,
My Mother.

In 1866, some sixty years after it first appeared, a learned professor of mathematics, Augustus De Morgan, wrote to *The Athenæum* describing the poem as 'one of the most beautiful lyrics in the English language'. But he took exception to the last verse, regarding it as 'a bit of religion thrust in'. He appealed, 'in the name of all the children of England', for the Poet Laureate, Tennyson, to be asked to supply an alternative version, unaware that Ann Taylor was still alive. Mrs Gilbert, as she then was, and in her eighties, replied, acknowledging that she would not now use the word 'vengeance' and herself offering the following alternative verse:

For could our Father in the skies
Look down with pleased or loving eyes,
If ever I could dare despise
My mother?

She did, however, make three points in her defence; that when she wrote the poem she was very young; that she still believed 'that all moral evil is sin'; and that in writing the last verse she was writing after the manner of Isaac Watts, 'our good old theologian'. De Morgan had raised the issue because he was so impressed by the poem, but his objection was to a tradition which he regarded as old-fashioned and without merit. Mrs Gilbert could recognise that she was out of step with the times, but for her the 'bit of religion' was the essence of her life (De Morgan, 1886; Armitage, 1939; Stewart, 1975; Darton, 1982).

The Taylor family and Ann and Jane's poetry for children has been introduced here at some length for two main reasons. First because they challenge prevailing mythologies about religiously inspired parenting; they cannot represent, but they are an example of a Puritan tradition of child-rearing that was far from repressive. Second, the fate of their poetry during the nineteenth century is an indication that in that period some of the most significant conflicts about childhood and about child-rearing appeared, conflicts that relate to religious and secular discourses which colour the whole development of childhood.

In the lives of the Taylor family, the conflicting conceptions of childhood innocence and evil perhaps found some kind of equilibrium, but around them and after them the intellectual and cultural maelstrom of the nineteenth century created a struggle about the nature of childhood, which was to infiltrate not only the everyday domestic scene, but also the public intellectual, literary and cultural life of the Victorian middle classes. There is a sense in which nineteenth-century conceptions of Puritanism will always be of more significance to us in the late twentieth century than will be the 'real' Puritans of the late sixteenth and seventeenth centuries. The reason for this lies in the force of Romanticism as a literary and cultural movement which intervened and began to make its impact at much the same time as Ann and Jane Taylor began to produce their poems.

Romanticism, as a cultural movement, must have a critical place in any discussion of childhood, not only because it shaped so many of our still powerful conceptions and, indeed, deepest feelings about children and about parenting, but also because, at the domestic and at the political level, it acquired its force in opposition not only to the growth of urban industrialism, but in opposition to the way in which religious evangelicism sought to shape child-rearing in the new industrialised society.

Nevertheless, there are good reasons for seeking a better understanding of the original Puritan experience. There is a simple debt to be paid to history, but beyond that it is difficult to understand what made the Puritan legacy so significant to the late eighteenth-century evangelical revival without understanding the intellectual and political context in which it struggled and briefly flourished. There is too a sense in which problems of child-rearing are existential and to examine the radical solutions which Puritanism offered has a value of its own which needs no further justification.

IN SEARCH OF THE 'REAL' PURITAN

What, then, of the original Puritans, of the late sixteenth and seventeenth centuries, who so irritated Elizabeth I, and who were later implicated in a revolution which saw the execution of Charles I? And what of those who left England in 1620 to found Plymouth Colony and those like John Winthrop who set up the flourishing colony in Massachusetts which really established New England? For those whose primary school history does allow them to venture back before the nineteenth century, another layer is added to the myth. The Puritan of the school textbook is the kill-joy who closed the theatres and publicly burned James I's *Book of Sports*, turning Sunday into a day of unrelieved constraint and tedium; he is the Roundhead of the civil war, with close cropped hair, dressed all in black except for the white collar (Unstead, 1955). Only slightly less unglamorous, he is one of those who, out of spite, sailed away upon the Mayflower; a hero of a muted kind, to be admired, perhaps, but not imitated.

It would be convenient to imagine that these layers of old cultural varnish could be stripped away to reveal Puritanism in its original form; that historians could provide us with the 'truth' about those families, parents and children, who have given rise to a myth of such enormous power. However, what we encounter, along with profound scholarship and ingenious research, is a number of historiographical controversies on which historians, themselves, must be left to adjudicate. It is interesting, for example, to note that Houlbrooke, in a standard text on the early modern family, covering the period 1450 to 1700, employs broad phrases such as 'pious Protestants' or 'Protestant Reformers', but rarely uses the term Puritan. This reflects, no doubt, the broad period he covers, but perhaps also an uncertainty about the value of Puritanism itself as a defining concept in relation to the family (Houlbrooke, 1984). Even so, taking account of the disagreements and the reticence these properly give rise to, there does seem to be a sense of Puritanism as a major social force within Protestantism, one which had considerable influence upon the way children were perceived and reared.

Sommerville has suggested that we should view Puritanism as a social movement; something which arises 'when change is apparent, when new possibilities are obvious, when disgust with old values becomes overpowering' (Sommerville, 1992: 12). In general terms a social movement can be described as follows. There emerge groups of people who share a general but identifiable set of aims and aspirations. They react against values which are seen as oppressive and irrelevant, seeing possibilities in the changes which take place in society but finding them frustratingly slow and partial. They try to develop a coherent ideology and to work out what practices this entails both in politics and in everyday life. In so doing they become objects of propaganda both of their supporters and of their detractors; the label their movement takes becomes both a symbol of progress and a term of abuse. The ideas and practices they generate are constrained by the dominant ideologies and social conventions of their day. But more radical groups may seek to break down or ignore these constraints, and in so doing (whilst they may have their moment) they are likely to be marginalised, especially by those who seek influence within the existing political and social institutions. If society as a whole changes direction, perhaps because of significant economic or political changes which destabilise society, then the movement might well find itself entering a much more introverted phase, in which a defence and perpetuation of its beliefs and practices require a more exclusive, more separatist way of life. Social movements, then, exist not as a set of beliefs, but as the social organisation which gives life to ideas. Puritanism was not a given set of dogmas which determined the way its adherents behaved, but a movement which faced a continual struggle to translate belief into practice.

Puritans were heirs of the Reformation, and part of the mainstream of Protestant thought and action, but they were 'restlessly critical and occasionally rebellious' in their desire to 'purify' the Church of England of its Papist origins (Hall quoted in Todd, 1987: 10). Theologically, their belief in the Calvinist doctrine of predestination did not set them apart from emerging Anglicanism until after 1620, when Archbishop Laud's espousal of Arminianism, with its emphasis upon grace attainable through the sacraments, reaffirmed the importance of ritual in religious observance. Laud's espousal of ritual and of a priestly hierarchy set him against the anti-clerical tendency of Puritans, their love of preaching and spreading of the Word (Stocker, 1992).

Politically, social reformers though they were, there was little to identify them as radical until they were made to appear so by the increasing authoritarianism and conservatism of pre-Civil War government (Todd, 1987). Puritanism provided a rallying cry, producing the inevitable backlash, as described by Lucy Hutchinson, the wife of Colonel Hutchinson of the Parliamentary Army.

> If any were grieved at the dishonour of the kingdom, or the griping of the pore, or the unjust oppression of the subject by a thousand ways invented to maintain the riots of the courtiers..., he was a Puritan;... if any gentleman in his country maintained the good laws of the land, or stood up for any public interest... for good order or government, he was a Puritan. In short all that crossed the interests of the needy courtiers, the proud encroaching priests... the lewd nobility and gentry... all these were Puritans.
>
> (quoted Hill, 1980: 90)

In the midst of the Civil War and during the ensuing Commonwealth, Puritans were radicalised by circumstance. Only the identification of the King with Antichrist could have justified regicide, but neither republicanism, nor democracy was part of their tradition. Indeed, most strove to distance themselves from the many more radical groups that sprang up, especially in the ranks of the victorious army. Nevertheless, the term 'enthusiast', used to condemn such extremists, was adopted after the Restoration in 1660 as a term with which to damn all dissenting groups. The Anglicanism that was established in 1660 after the restoration of Charles II sought to define itself in opposition to the religious practices of the Commonwealth and hence set out to 'demonise Puritanism as that which had overthrown monarchy' (Stocker, 1992: 54).

Thus neither in political nor religious terms did Puritans control their own destiny, except possibly those who had taken the decision to leave the country of their birth and seek a place free from corruption in New England. Even such a dramatic venture was not without its difficulties, however, and corruption in the form of what Edmund Morgan calls a 'horde of average, lusty Elizabethan Englishmen' pursued them across the Atlantic, but at least the colonists were not caught in the political maelstrom which engulfed mid-seventeenth-century England (Morgan, 1966: 170). It is not surprising, therefore, even when what is under discussion concerns the private rather than the public sphere, that the historiography of Puritanism should be influenced by the dramatic nature of seventeenth-century politics. To some extent this is entirely appropriate and it is undoubtedly true that Puritans, when they preached and wrote endlessly about questions relating to marriage and child-rearing, saw in the family a microcosm of church and state.

HISTORICAL ACCOUNTS OF PURITANISM

The revolutionary political context of the seventeenth century has tended to produce a view of the Puritans as also revolutionary within the domestic sphere. Indeed, in its classic formulation in the work of Christopher Hill, the revolutionary nature of the Puritans spreads to the economic sphere as well, linking them to the rising bourgeoisie through their commitment to work and hostility to idleness. Through their efforts the stagnant, inefficient feudal economy began its transformation to a modern capitalist one. Hill finds in the Puritans (to use a seventeenth-century phrase) 'an industrious sort of people' who attributed the undeveloped nature of the seventeenth-century English economy to the idleness of labour. For the Puritans labour became a social duty, incumbent upon women as well as men, and thrift a virtue. Such a doctrine could have a radical edge to it when applied not only to the poor but also to the idle rich (Hill, 1964).

Central to Hill's account is the 'spiritualisation of the household' which placed the broader family, including apprentices and servants, at the centre of moral, political and economic life; a little commonwealth, the 'lowest unit in the hierarchy of discipline', as Hill puts it (1964: 443). The increased importance of the household as the basic economic unit produced a strongly patriarchal society. The symbolic significance of women may have declined with the decreasing religious significance of the Saints and especially of the Virgin Mary, but the marriage of priests under Protestantism may have elevated the status of women as marriage partners. As mothers, too, they acquired a higher profile as mediators of patriarchal authority to female servants and, of course, to their children.

Such an account presents Puritanism as a significant element in the modernising process which was already driving English society in the direction of industrialisation and towards the modern, bourgeois social order we associate with it. Not least striking in Hill's account is the intellectual vigour of Puritanism; the almost obsessive desire to write, to discuss and to argue. So that, for example, advice about domestic conduct in the many books devoted to this topic is not the mere delineation of proper etiquette but is concerned to regulate behaviour according to a moral view of the whole social order. Hill's account is relatively untainted by nineteenth-century perceptions of Puritan child-rearing practices; indeed, he refers to 'the slow but significant humanisation of relations between parents and children which took place in the sixteenth and seventeenth centuries', and there is no doubting his general admiration for what he sees as the revolutionary energy of Puritanism (Hill, 1964: 453).

Lawrence Stone's view of the domestic influence of the Puritans is, on the other hand, equivocal. This is not because of any naive Romantic vision, however, but rather because Stone is concerned to trace a linear development in domestic relations from a state of mutual indifference to one of 'affective individualism'. The late sixteenth and seventeenth centuries witnessed a transition from one state to the other, and hence the Puritan movement stands between them, looking forward in terms of emotional intensity, but having not yet found the respect for individuals that, according to Stone, began to emerge only in the later seventeenth and eighteenth centuries (Stone, 1977).

For Stone the spiritualisation of the household did, indeed, lead to an intense interest in children, a greatly increased concern for their welfare and to a warmer, more intense mother–child relationship. But since the object of parenting was the development of inner discipline in the child, mothering, especially, was also a desperately serious business.

> Many late sixteenth and seventeenth century mothers were both caring and repressive at the same time for the simple reason that the two went together. Puritans in particular were profoundly concerned about their children, loved them and subjected them to endless moral pressure. At the same time they feared and even hated them as agents of sin within the household, and therefore beat them mercilessly.
>
> (Stone 1979: 125)

In Stone's account, Puritanism is lodged within a broader process of change between 1500 and 1700 which witnessed the decline of authority of kinship in the face of the growing power of the nation state as well as the 'missionary success of Protestantism, especially its Puritan wing, in bringing Christian morality to a majority of homes'

(Stone, 1975: 13). Stone finds in Puritanism the origins of a disciplinary society, at the centre of which stood the nuclear family, emotionally intense, looking out to wider society in its proselytising zeal, but anxiously concerned with its own internal discipline, a focus for 'psychological loyalty and devotion' (ibid.: 25). Love within marriage was emphasised, he says, but so was the authority of the male head of the household and the status of women declined. Stone believes there is broad evidence of a much harsher treatment of children, especially in schools but also within the home where the utmost respect was demanded by both parents, a respect which did not diminish with adulthood. Even in their forties 'Gentlemen of thirty or forty years old were to stand like mutes and fools bareheaded before their parents' (Aubrey, quoted ibid.: 41). Daughters, even those who had become the wives of peers, still knelt in their mother's presence. Such deference was established, according to Stone, by an upbringing in which child-rearing was equated 'with the breaking in of young horses or hunting dogs' (ibid.: 37).

Behind this severe approach to child-rearing lay the religious fears of parents for the future salvation of their offspring and Stone finds in this a paradoxical response to a growing interest in children. According to Stone, this interest was first manifested as a celebration of childhood innocence and purity in the Italian Renaissance, but the moral thrust of the Protestant Reformation twisted it into a 'deadly fear of the liability of children to corruption and sin, particularly those cardinal sins of pride and disobedience' (ibid.: 43). At its most extreme, this fear led Calvin to advocate the death penalty for disobedience to parents, a precept actually translated into legislation in parts of New England in the 1640s, though never, as far as is known, acted upon. Stone also sees a non-religious motivation behind parents' severity, especially in upper-class circles, since the achievement of docile subordination in childhood would increase the economic control of parents when it came to later critical questions of marriage and career. He also notes that the spread of education at home as well as in schools necessitated a greater control of children. The tedium of the Renaissance education diet of Latin and Greek cannot have helped, as John Locke was to point out with some force at the end of the seventeenth century.

What Stone does is to relate what he believes to be the increasingly harsh treatment of children in the sixteenth and seventeenth centuries to political and economic as well as to religious causes. He sees this as a transitional phase between the kin-orientated, psychically numb pre-Reformation world, and the modern world of affective and tolerant domestic relationships. Though Stone does not distinguish a specifically Puritan mode of child-rearing, Puritanism provides him with the archetype for his transitional model, the 'restricted, patriarchal, nuclear family'. Religion, education, politics (and perhaps evolving capitalist economics, though Stone makes less of this than Hill) bring to bear upon the child conflicting forces. On the one hand an *intention* towards modernity, but on the other the *methods* of the old world; a disciplined, educated child to be reared through strict religious precepts and an irrelevant curriculum.

Stone's work has been much criticised. Its scope is alarming, and its use of evidence selective. The focus is too much upon the upper echelons of society to reveal much about even the middling ranks. The narrative, however sophisticated, remains Whiggish, a story of human progress (Macfarlane, 1979; Gillis, 1979; Thompson, 1977). Nevertheless, his ideas are attractive precisely because he combines the myth of the repressed, religious childhood, represented to the twentieth century by the Victorians, with a historical tradition which finds the origins of modern western society in the very period of British and American history when Puritanism was at its most influential. By a very ingenious, if ultimately unsatisfactory, manipulation of myth, recent historiography and copious if selective evidence, Stone allows us to keep both our traditional distaste for Puritan child-rearing and yet grant them a not unpalatable motivation for their allegedly repressive practices.

Two main lines of criticism have emerged in relation to the approach of Hill and Stone to Puritanism. The first of these is directed against the view of the Puritans as a radical, revolutionary force. As Todd, one of Hill's critics, puts it,

> Hill and his followers have Puritan social thought rising phoenix-like from the ashes of medieval social and intellectual stagnation to ignite the Civil War and usher in a new bourgeois social system in seventeenth century England.
>
> (Todd, 1987: 4)

We have already noted that Puritanism emerged out of mainstream Protestantism, and was forced during the course of the seventeenth century into opposition to Anglicanism. But there were also influences beyond Protestantism. Commentators such as Houlbrooke, for example, find echoes from pre-Reformation writers (Houlbrooke 1984: 156). Indeed, Schucking, writing in the 1920s, had already suggested indigenous origins dating from the Middle Ages, as well as Protestant influences, for what he called the 'pietistic family community', with its emphasis upon the education of the young and its characteristic reverence for Sunday (Schucking, 1969: 59). The search for the origins of Puritan social thought has been recently undertaken most systematically by Todd. She argues that the origins of the 'spiritualisation of the household' can be found in the humanism of Catholic writers like Erasmus, Vives and Thomas More (Todd, 1980: 19).

For Todd an emphasis upon early religious education, upon the significance of the mother's role, upon the extreme deference due from child to parent, and upon the importance of reasoning with the child – all these are to be found in Catholic writers. The division between Protestantism and Catholicism, Todd attributes to the Counter-Reformation, and in particular to the threat the Council of Trent saw in household religious education, a threat to the authority of the priest. Hence the post-Tridentine Catholic authorities gave to bishops, not to fathers and mothers, responsibility for catechising the young (ibid.: 33). Todd does not seek to minimise the significance of Puritan influence upon domestic social thought, but she sees Puritans as effective propagandists for, rather than as originators of, the ideas they tried to put into practice; these had their origins in the Renaissance rather than in the Reformation. Puritans were self-conscious reformers who, at least until the upheavals that presaged the Civil War, worked as zealots within a broader Protestant tradition. As evangelists they were identifiable by others and by themselves as a people who had a distinct view of how the world should be, who tried both to preach its virtues to others and put it into practice themselves (Todd, 1987).

The second line of criticism, has been directed particularly at harsh, pessimistic judgements of Puritan child-rearing practices in particular. In seeing Puritan attitudes to child-rearing as a perversion of some emerging Renaissance ideal, Stone presents them in their worst light, but others have taken a less critical view. Houlbrooke, for example, sees a tension between, 'Protestant writers' pessimistic premises concerning human nature, and their relatively liberal practical advice concerning upbringing, influenced by classical and humanist precepts' (Houlbrooke, 1984: 143). But for Houlbrooke this led to moderation not excess, to a search for a balance between severity and indulgence and to a sense of the complexity of the business of rearing children, and of the 'fine judgment' needed to succeed. Stone finds children treated with extreme severity, parents beating their children without mercy for the sake of their souls. Clearly he regards this as the norm, but Edmund Morgan can find no proof that seventeenth-century New England parents were any more likely than twentieth-century parents to resort to corporal punishment, for example (Morgan, 1966: 103). Linda Pollock, in her extensive examination of diaries and autobiographies, fails to find, for either the sixteenth or the seventeenth centuries, evidence of widespread corporal punishment, and no systematic evidence to suggest that Puritan parents stood out in any way (Pollock, 1983). John Morgan too concludes that use of the rod was regarded as a sign of failure on the part of parents, its final justification lying only in the fear of eternal damnation (Morgan, 1986: 149). The most recent attempt to rescue Puritans from the charge of general beastliness comes from Sommerville, who claims to find in Puritan writing not only a realistic view of the nature of childhood (and, by implication, a realistic view of the response parents should make), but also a sense of humour and of realism in their approach to children (Sommerville, 1992).

THE PURITAN 'PLAN-FOR-ACTION'

What this discussion of the historiographical debate illustrates is the difficulty of finding a way of approaching Puritans, their beliefs and behaviour. Sommerville has referred to a general failure in childhood studies to distinguish between social and cultural histories, between the lived experience of a particular group at a particular time, and the process of cultural formation which informs but also inhibits and determines behaviour (Sommerville, 1992: 3). As the methodologies of cultural and social history develop, so the grand theories of a Christopher Hill or a Lawrence Stone look increasingly vulnerable. It also becomes more difficult to choose a point of entry into an increasingly fragmented historical discourse (Hunt, 1989).

One potentially fruitful approach is to look more carefully at the internal dynamics of Puritan thought about the family. That will allow us to understand both why readings of evidence as varied as those of Stone and Sommerville are possible, and also to explore the possibility that external factors impinging upon the Puritan movement in both England and America affected the Puritan approach to domestic life.

Even at this abstract level of ideas, we should not, as John Morgan points out, look for too tidy a picture, too coherent an exposition. Not only did Puritans frequently disagree with each other, but their ideas were generated in a specific context; ideas and context conflicting to produce programmes for action which were a compromise. As Morgan says, 'There is . . . a continuum of intellectual action, from first conceptions and intellectual influences all the way through to the commission of an act based (in part) upon one's principles and beliefs'. Morgan himself seeks to explore 'the ways in which . . . ideas could be connected to *intention* in social action . . . the connexion between principle and plan-for-action' (Morgan, 1986: 6).

Given the Puritan belief in predestination, many commentators have asked themselves why Puritans were so concerned with this earthly life and particularly with the education of their children. Indeed their scorn for 'civil man', the man who outwardly lived a virtuous life, was intense. Thomas Shepard, one of the first ministers of the Puritan churches created in Massachusetts, New England, in the 1630s thundered accordingly:

> What though thy life be smooth, what though thy outside, thy sepulchre, be painted? O, thou art full of rottenness, of sin, within. Guilty, not before men, as the sins of thy life make thee, but before God, of all the sins that swarm and roar in the whole world at this day, for God looks to the heart; guilty thou art therefore of heart whoredom, heart sodomy, heart blasphemy, heart drunkenness, heart buggery, heart oppression, heart idolatry; and these are the sins that terribly provoke the wrath of Almighty God against thee.
>
> (quoted in Morgan, 1966: 1)

Edmund Morgan has suggested that Puritans justified social virtue on the grounds that, though salvation was not possible through a virtuous life (how could anybody believe that they could justify themselves to God), yet virtue was a necessary way for the elect, those chosen by God, to maintain their belief in their own salvation. Furthermore, since all sin was to be opposed, virtue was to be imposed upon others, and especially by the Puritan father and householder upon his family and household. This special commitment to the family derived from God's covenant with Abraham, which was a promise not only to Abraham, but to his seed for ever. Hence there was a special relationship between father and children on the question of salvation, and more broadly between one generation and the next.

John Morgan goes further and argues that, for English Puritans especially, the *pursuit* of salvation became the 'basis for a coherent religious and social ethic' (Morgan, 1986: 24). Good works and a blameless life were not on their own sufficient, but, together with continual repentance for one's sins, they offered the best guide to the assurance of salvation. Each person had to wait until they were offered the covenant by God, but they could prepare themselves for the event and ensure that they were ready for it by learning to examine the state of their own soul. God, too, might listen to those who earnestly sought him.

Puritans experienced the pull of two contradictory forces. The doctrine of predestination could lead to antinomianism, to a belief that the 'elect' were above any obligation to adhere to moral laws propounded by mere mortals, to believe that they had, as it were, a direct line to God. It was, however, one thing to cite Scripture in argument with fellow Puritans, but another to claim direct revelation from God Himself. In any case, predestination was a complex doctrine even for an educated elite (Doran and Durston, 1991). In striving to bring a congregation to an appreciation of its responsibilities, both spiritual and worldly, there was an inevitable tendency to over-emphasise the efficacy of works as against the absolute necessity for faith, to speak too much of the merit of human actions, rather than of the grace of God. The Arminian theology of Archbishop Laud was not easily excluded from the everyday practice of Puritanism.

Arminianism may also have caused problems other than those strictly associated with theology, in that Laud's desire to enhance the 'beauty of holiness' lead him to re-assert the importance of ceremonial and ritual in religious practice. The Puritan response came not only through the iconophobia of the mid-seventeenth century that has left such a powerful impression upon our folk image of Puritanism, but in the more general Protestant emphasis upon close scriptural exegesis. As recent scholars have emphasised, this rational approach to religion and ethics was, for the educated Puritan, by no means confined to the study of scripture but followed in the footsteps of the Christian humanists in using classical sources (Todd, 1987). Nevertheless, reason had its limits and John Morgan shows how they were caught between a belief in justification by faith alone and the attraction of the humanist belief in human learning. On the one side was enthusiasm and fervency, the desire to search one's soul through prayer and endless self-examination; on the other was a belief that ceremonial and ritual were signs of papist corruption, and that God had to be sought through the exercise of the mind (Morgan, 1986: 64).

When the Puritan Minister Ralph Josselin's daughter Mary lay dying in May of 1669, he opened his Bible at random, letting the pages fall open where they would. He was seeking through scripture some words of comfort from God, some message that would touch his heart and comfort him. An educated man, Josselin translated the despised rituals of Roman Catholicism into his own private search for God's meaning. So he took the Bible, the principal source for any rational explanation of God's purpose, and turned it into a talisman, an almost magical symbol of the presence of God in his life. In this he probably acted as many of his fellow Puritans did.

Puritans experienced another sort of tension in knowing how much they should be part of the world in which they found themselves and how far they should separate themselves from its failures and inadequacies. Those who sailed on the *Mayflower*, for example, were separatists who sought to protect themselves from the corruption that oppressed them. On the other hand, John Winthrop, before he sailed from England in 1630, agonised over whether he was justified in deserting his country, even though he saw it sliding further and further into sin. In Massachusetts, he spent much of his life as governor, striving to prevent separatist zeal from fragmenting the mission of creating a godly society (Morgan, 1958).

This godly society for which Puritans aimed was both hierarchical and patriarchal. The impact that Puritanism had upon women is ambiguous. Whilst within the household, the authority of the husband was absolute, the role of the wife, not least in taking responsibility for the education of young children, was probably enhanced. In any case the final commitment was to God and not to husband; the authority of the husband was shaped by external constraints of religious principle, as well as by duty and love (Morgan, 1958: 13). Both were to play their role within a framework which prescribed precise duties and responsibilities. Clearly, however, household circumstances would affect the way in which household relationships were worked out. In a household like that of Ralph Josselin where, although a minister, Josselin was around the house a great deal and both husband and wife worked together on the farm, something approaching a companionate marriage probably existed in which the bringing up of the children, especially, was a shared responsibility (Macfarlane, 1970: 115). On the other hand, in the case of John Winthrop, frequently away from home and preoccupied with public affairs, his wife Margaret must have shaped her role in the shadow of her husband's public duties, and with an acceptance of the different parts allotted by God to man and wife.

This is not the place to elaborate upon the general status of women within Puritanism, except to say that, in Puritan writing, their status as mothers seems to have been more secure than their status as wives (Leverenz, 1980). Perhaps more immediately important to children than the relative status of husband and wife was the different roles of father and mother. More than one commentator has noted that in their writings Puritans tend to talk of 'parents', when not talking specifically of the mothering of infants, implying joint involvement (Leverenz, 1980: 80; Todd, 1987: 105). Both Demos, specifically in relation to the separatist Plymouth Colony, and Leverenz more generally, have argued for a sharp contrast between the earlier years when mothering was intense, loving and far from repressive, and the later years of childhood and adolescence when 'tender mothering' was replaced by the guidance of the father as a 'grave governor' (Demos, 1970; Leverenz, 1980).

Perhaps of particular significance is the pervasiveness of the image of mothering in Puritan writing. Leverenz, in particular, has noted the way in which female images of God as a 'nursing Father' and of ministers as the 'breasts of God' nourishing their congregations are common in Puritan sermons. It has a parallel too in the insistence of the domestic conduct books upon the importance of breast feeding; William Gouge could find well over twenty reasons why mothers should breast feed their babies. Fathers, too, come to share the nursing imagery; they should be longing to impart their knowledge 'as a Nurse to empty her breasts' (Leverenz, 1980: 72). Nor was the imagery confined to the nursing duties of mothers. Thus, John Cotton, one of the ministers to leave for New England in the 1630s, told his congregation

> Women, if they were not Mothers, would not take such homely offices up, as to cleanse their Children from their filth; why if God were not of the like affection to us, he would not cleanse us from our filthiness... it is with us as it is with young Infants that would lie in their defilements, if their Mothers did not make them clean, and so would wee even wallow in the defilements of sin, if God did not cleanse us, therefore admire God's love and mercy towards us.
>
> (quoted Leverenz, 1980: 124)

Few would now accept Stone's pessimistic view of Puritan repressiveness. Extreme examples can always be found, but most commentators stress the insistence of Puritan writers upon the virtue of finding a balance between love and discipline. Certainly they expressed great fears over excessive 'cockering' of young children and were continually fearful lest love for their children should lead parents to neglect their duty. But equally, they deplored the use of physical punishment, regarding it as counter-productive, to be used only as a last resort.

Perhaps, as Leverenz suggests, the real (and more natural) fear was of the rebellious adolescent. Bunyan would certainly have seemed to have thought so in his poem 'Upon the Disobedient Child':

> Children become, while little, our delights
> When they grow bigger, they begin to fright's.
>
> They take the Counsels of a Wanton's rather
> Than the most grave Instructions of a Father.
>
> But wretched child, how canst thou thus requite
> Thy Aged Parents, for that great delight
> They took in thee, when thou, as helpless lay
> In their Indulgent Bosoms day by day?
>
> But now, behold, how they rewarded are!
> For their Indulgent Love, and Tender Care,
> All is forgot, this love he doth despise
> They brought this bird up to peck out their Eyes.
>
> (Midgely, 1980)

The dynamics of Puritan child-rearing were infinitely more complex than would be suggested by Victorian mythology. To establish the child's obedience to parents and to all sources of legitimate authority was the immediate aim of Puritan parenting. Initially girls and boys could learn from their mothers the virtue both of authority and of submissiveness; for girls, mothers could continue to be a role model, whilst boys would have to model themselves upon their fathers. But the ultimate aim of parents was to bring their children to conversion, to a state where they could respond to the call from God when it came. To do this the will of the child, which existed long before the advent of reason, had to be denied. But the justification for this denial was not repressive, but to ensure that the child learned the necessity of self-denial and the development of a godly conscience. Original sin was not, as Edmund Morgan points out, 'a fairy story with which to frighten little children', it was a fact of life. It had to be fought with both education and discipline. Puritan ministers urged early religious education, because the earlier sin was combatted, the better the chance of victory. Hence when their children woke, when they went to bed, when they ate and when they played, parents were encouraged to instruct them (Morgan, 1966: 96). More formal instruction came through the catechism, in which children learned by rote the answers to questions of religious belief and practice. What was learned by rote in early childhood was built upon by school and by the minister, in order to lead the growing child to the Bible, the only true source of godly knowledge (Morgan, 1986: 155).

Knowledge on its own was not sufficient, however. Nor was self-denial unless it lead to fervency, to an overwhelming desire to repent of a sinful nature and seek assurance of salvation from God. Discipline and self-denial were to lead not only to a receptiveness to instruction, but to an inner conviction of the sinfulness of human nature. To remind a child of its mortality was to concentrate the mind upon the ever pressing need for obedience, to emphasise the need to act as a saint, even before the vital moment of conversion finally brought the assurance of salvation.

Hence the aim of Puritan parenting was awesome, and awesome it must have appeared to many children, but it went beyond the simple demand for obedience. Salvation was the ultimate aim, and with it the ecstasy that the assurance of salvation could bring to the saints. The *method*, therefore, was to be as gentle as possible. 'Repression', John Morgan remarks, 'was obviously not the spiritual equal of conversion' (Morgan, 1986: 149). Much advice to parents stresses the importance of the middle way, since only by persuasion could the child learn, not only to fear damnation, but the anticipated joys of salvation. To be effective, furthermore, teaching had to suit not only the general limitations of childhood, but also the individuality of each child. The poet Anne Bradstreet, herself the mother of eight children, used the metaphor of flesh needing salt as a preservative and fruit sugar, to describe the diversity of children's needs. She concluded, 'those parents are wise that can fit their nurture according to their Nature' (quoted Morgan, 1966: 107).

Perhaps one of Janeway's stories can capture the experience of Puritan childhood better than anything. Not in the sense of being typical or representative, but rather in the way that Janeway captures, through the confrontation of the child with death, a sense of the emotional intensity, the fervency that both the search for and the experience of the assurance of salvation could bring. The story of Sarah Howley opens with her being awakened to her sinful condition by a sermon. Her response is immediate:

> She wept bitterly to think what a case she was in; and went home, and got herself into a chamber, and upon her knees she wept and cried to the Lord as well as she could, which might easily be perceived by her eyes and countenance.

Another sermon intensifies her feelings so that 'she could scarce speak of sin, or be spoke to, but her heart was ready to melt', and she seeks solace in reading scripture and other books which direct her to make religion the focus of her life. This manifests itself first of all in her attitude to her parents:

> She was exceeding dutiful to her parents, very loath to grieve them in the least: And if she had at any time (which was very rare) offended them, she would weep bitterly.

She abhors lying, spends her time conscientiously, working diligently at school and becoming eminent for her 'teachableness, meekness and modesty'. Whilst in this state she becomes fatally ill and once more very fearful of her soul. She begs her mother to pray for her, 'That I may have a saving knowledge of sin and Christ, and that I may have an assurance of God's love to my soul.' Most of all she fears she will deceive herself into believing she is saved and when her father tries to reassure her that she is going to a 'better father' she falls into a passion:

> but how do I know that I am a poor sinner that wants assurance. O for assurance! It was still her note. O for assurance! This was her great earnest and constant request to all that came to her, to beg assurance for her; and, poor heart, she would look with so much eagerness upon them, as if she desired nothing in the world so much as that they would pity her, and help her with their prayers; never was poor creature more earnest for any thing than she was for an assurance and the light of God's countenance. O the piteous moan that she would make! O the agonies that her soul was in.

All the neighbourhood pray for her as she finally learns to wait in patience for God's assurance, venturing her soul upon Christ. Eventually, her prayers are answered and she is filled with divine rapture:

> Lord, thou hast promised, that whosoever comes unto thee, thou wilt in no wise cast out; Lord, I come unto thee, and surely thou wilt in no wise cast me out. O so sweet: O so glorious is Jesus! O I have the sweet and glorious Jesus; he is sweet, he is sweet, he is sweet! O the admirable love of God in sending Christ! O free grace to a poor lost creature.

Now she longs for death to take her to Jesus, but she attempts, as she dies, to warn her brothers and sisters to make their calling and election sure while they are still in health:

> O if you knew how good Christ were! O if you had but one taste of his sweetness, you would rather go to him a thousand times, than stay in this wicked world. I would not for ten thousand and ten thousand worlds part with my interest in Christ.

This is the intense, heightened, emotional world of Janeway but the immediacy of a child's relationship with God is also brought home by Josselin's diary account of his little 5-year-old daughter Jane, who

> dreamed that Jesus Christ was in our church, and went up to my pulpit, and there stayed a while, and then he came down, and came to bed with her. She said to him, 'Why dost thou come to me', and he answered her, 'To sleep a little with thee' and he layed down and slept, and again she dreamed that Jesus Christ told her that he should come and reign upon the earth 1,000 years (Feb. 5th, 1651).
> (Macfarlane, 1976)

The task of Puritan parents (and beyond them the wider world of adults) was to represent to their children both the awesome power of God and his infinite love, to bring Christ into the dreams of their young offspring both as one who might sleep beside them and as a king who would reign for a thousand years.

It is inevitably difficult to disentangle a distinctively Puritan approach to child-rearing. As Todd has shown, their approach to education and even to the spiritualisation of the household, was by no means unique to them. The fact that Puritanism, as a social movement, was engaged for a period of over a hundred years in dramatic political events is no guarantee that domestic experience was equally dramatic. Imprisoning an archbishop, executing a king, even emigrating across the Atlantic, does not of itself disturb the underlying continuities of family life. Durston, in his study of the seventeenth-century English family, finds examples from Ralph Josselin's diary of an over-riding preoccupation with the family. For example, on 12 July 1654, Josselin notes that the day was set aside for the election of members to Cromwell's first Protectorate Parliament, but adds 'and I set it apart to seek god in behalf of my family'. Later, on reporting a rumour that Cromwell was to be proclaimed Emperor, Josselin adds to the same sentence 'God good in preserving Ann in a milk bowl, and Jane from swooning, who let her fall in' (quoted Durston, 1989: 172).

True, there could be stormy controversies over religious rituals associated with childhood. For example over the churching of women after childbirth, and, especially, both in New and Old England, over infant baptism. The mainstream Puritans of New England maintained it along with the Lord's Supper as the only two sacraments, and it caused considerable difficulties in knowing whose children should be baptised. Should baptism be confined only to the children of those who were fully received into the church, the body of the elect whose offspring were of the seed of Abraham; or should it be extended to the children of any baptised person, whether or not they were accepted as one of the saints? More liberal factions wanted the baptismal sacrament extended even further (Bremer, 1976: 144).

In England the outbreak of Civil War brought the question of infant baptism into prominence. John and Lucy Hutchinson decided, after careful thought and consultation of the Bible and of ministers, not to have their child, born in 1646, baptised. For their pains they were treated as fanatics by their fellow worshippers. Attempts to change the rituals of baptism and to abolish godparents seem not to have gone down too well; public ceremonies declined, but private baptisms may have become more common. Upon the establishment of the post-Restoration Anglican church, it seems to have been with a sense of relief that Ralph Josselin and his congregation settled down to the old pre-Revolution practices (Durston, 1989: 121).

PURITAN CHILD-REARING OVER TIME

Such public controversies and conflicts tell us something about day-to-day child-rearing practices, but our knowledge of the actual lives of Puritan families remains sketchy. The same is true of the way in which these practices changed over time, to the way in which the 'plan-for-action' was affected by changing circumstances. Furthermore there is a danger in assuming that the influences were in one direction, that is from theology to child-rearing practices. For example, in his book, *The Puritan Family*, Edmund Morgan examines the impact Puritanism had upon the family, but he seeks also to inquire 'whether the natural relationships between husband and wife and between parents and children did not influence the way Puritans thought about God and the church' (Morgan, 1966: 161). Morgan points out the extent to which Puritan theology is expressed in domestic terms, and though at one level, this is no more than metaphor, yet the representation is so powerful as to suggest that 'Puritan's religious experiences in some way duplicated their domestic experiences' (ibid.: 166); God was recreated through Puritan language into a more domestic Being. In this way Puritans claimed God as their own, a tribal deity as Morgan has it, and they claimed Him not only for themselves, but especially for their children. As the Puritan experiment in New England faltered and was increasingly exposed to the influence of the ungodly, so, Morgan suggests, their tribalism increased. As their children deserted the tribe, they failed to seek new blood from outside, but instead strove with even greater intensity to keep their own offspring. Thus Increase Mather, a second generation New England minister, painted a dismal picture of the last Day:

> when a Child shall see his Father at the right Hand of Christ in the day of Judgment but himself at His left Hand: And when his Father shall joyn with Christ in passing a Sentence of Eternal Death upon him, saying, Amen O Lord, thou art Righteous in thus Judging: And when after the Judgment, children shall see their Father going with Christ to Heaven, but themselves going into Everlasting Punishment.
>
> (quoted ibid.: 179)

In the developing, economically prosperous, but socially fragmenting colonies of New England, a degree of defensiveness was inevitable, but the tensions inherent in the Puritan doctrine of predestination may have made child-rearing an increasingly anxious process. Neither rigorous intellectual preparation for the godly life, nor intense evangelical appeals to the emotions could, as Morgan says, guarantee that children would experience conversion, that 'final ecstatic experience of grace without which true devotion must prove impossible' (ibid.: 185). Morgan is severe in his judgement, accusing Puritans of committing the sin of placing their children higher than God in their affections. 'When theology became the handmaid of genealogy,' he concludes, 'Puritanism no longer deserved its name' (ibid.: 186).

Sommerville finds a not dissimilar process taking place in England itself. After the oppressions of the 1630s, the Civil War and the subsequent Commonwealth opened up possibilities for Puritanism, which were to be dashed with the Restoration and the establishment of the Anglican church. Thus the broad Puritan movement which had been able to operate, if not without difficulty, within the mainstream of Protestantism, was branded as traitorous, at least until the Toleration Act of 1689. For Sommerville, this experience turned Puritanism from broad social movement to sect. Post-Restoration Dissenters fell back upon the family and turned inward, and as a consequence became more obsessive and oppressive in their child-rearing.

For Sommerville it is less the conjunction of theology and circumstance that produces this effect and more the result of persecution (Sommerville, 1992: 15). Sommerville appears to be looking for the origin of the Victorian myth of the repressive Puritan parent and discovering it in the Restoration persecution of non-conformity. Thus the introverted, threatened family implodes with the result that the Puritan sense of balance, the middle way, in parenting is lost.

A more elaborate theory is expounded by Leverenz which bears some relationship to Morgan's. Like Morgan, Leverenz is acutely sensitive to the language of Puritan writing. He sees literary sources (mostly sermons and instructional tracts) as particularly valuable because through them he believes the repressed feelings of collective Puritanism were expressed (Leverenz, 1980: 18). All social movements depend upon the development of a language through which shared significances are created and propagated. Such languages are representations of the beliefs, attitudes and practices of the members of that movement. All representations have to be understood in relation to their particular mode of expression; they are not mere mirrors of reality. Most of the evidence we have of human behaviour is mediated through languages of representation.

Whilst the actual behaviour of Puritan families may elude us, not least because generalisation is so hazardous, they have bequeathed us a rich archive of linguistic representation. It is this that Leverenz explores. Morgan, we have noted, identified the linguistic domestication of the Puritan God, and we have already referred to Leverenz's own discussion of the overwhelming intensity of the imagery of mothering in Puritan writing. Thus, in the language of Puritan writing, religion and the family fuse. The imagery of mothering, intensely, almost passionately loving, tender and nurturing, gave some legitimacy to female weakness, paralleled in God's weakness, His extreme forbearance for sinful humanity. Mothers, suggests Leverenz, using Winnicot's phrase, could be 'good enough' (Leverenz, 1980: 79). But as at the Last Day God's judgement would be unforgiving, so the father took ultimate responsibility for his family. The 'grave governor' of the household was allowed no weakness, his authority gave him duties and responsibilities, but no respite in dependency. Yet as a human being, he would no doubt fail at times, and as a sinner seeking the assurance of salvation, he would be for ever dependent upon the grace of God. Thus, suggests Leverenz, the intertwining of a loving yet wrathful God with images of the parental roles meant that 'The Puritan Family was sending a pervasive mixed signal to its young: feel nourished and valued, yet feel sinful and ashamed' (Leverenz, 1980: 100).

Leverenz, too, like Morgan and Sommerville, believes that over time the dynamics of Puritan parenting led to a growing introversion. He suggests no external force, but describes a process created by the psychological forces inherent in the Puritan parenting. These forces led to the overwhelming of mothering by the guilt-ridden and fearful fathering. One concrete and observable result of this, Leverenz believes, was that breaking the will was attempted earlier, and there are eighteenth-century examples of evangelical parents attempting to break the wills of very young infants (Greven, 1977). As conversion experiences amongst young adults declined, so parents became more anxious and in their anxiety encouraged younger and younger children to have conversion experiences.

Here, in the reborn child, captured, as we have seen, in the emotional religiosity of James Janeway's *A Token for Children*, is the beginning of a fantasy about childhood innocence that lasted far into the nineteenth century. Indeed, as Sommerville notes, there are suggestions of 'natural' piety in some of Janeway's children, who might therefore appear to have no need of conversion (Sommerville, 1992: 55). There would be a curious irony if, in the days of Puritan confusion and the beginnings of the identification of Puritanism with excessively repressive parenting, the child of mystical innocence also made its first appearance. The long-term effect upon parenting, suggests Leverenz, was that with the increasing separation of the father from the household (and hence from its spirituality), and the growing power of the mother within it as the sole arbiter of morality, the lingering image of paternal severity becomes divorced from the everyday language and practice of the family. The extraordinary linguistic intertwining of God and parenting is lost.

THE IMAGE OF PURITANISM

This story of growing introversion is attractive, not least because, by adding a historical dimension to the analysis, it suggests how Puritan parenting might have changed during the course of the seventeenth century both in New and in Old England. Especially seductive is the explanation it offers for the discrepancy between the progressive aspects of parenting now generally accepted to be part of the message of Elizabethan and early seventeenth-century Puritanism and the harsh judgement of Victorian Romanticism.

Nevertheless, the theory of Puritan radicalism refuses to die, not least because the economic theory of Puritans as being at the forefront of the development of economic capitalism and political individualism also refuses to die. Most recently Sommerville has seen in Puritanism one stage in a long process of conflict between the individual and the family. Inherent in Puritan theology, he suggests, is a profound individualism, embodied in the relationship between the individual and their God. But because Puritans could not cope with the consequences this had for the family, they compromised and through covenant theology tried to grant their own children a special place. This in turn increased the pressure upon Puritan parents to ensure the conversion of their children. Thus the family gained its victory over the individual, and parenting became more anxious and oppressive. But, claims Sommerville, the force of individualism did not die, it resurfaced in the political radicalism of the late eighteenth century, especially in the writings of William Godwin, who fiercely attacked the family as an obstacle to freedom and reform (Sommerville, 1992).

Individualism, however, is too protean a concept to bear the weight of such an explanation. To say that the family is in conflict with the individual is a mere truism unless the nature of that conflict can be more precisely stated. There is force in argument that covenant theology was an accommodation of belief to the force of familial loyalties – Edmund Morgan, too, uses the same argument – but the nature of Puritan individualism is harder to detect. Perhaps most vividly, it was to be found in the anxious self-analysis that was manifested in the emphasis upon prayer and in the writing of diaries as private reckonings of an individual's standing with the Almighty.

But it is difficult to see how this introverted response to the guilt of sinfulness should arise after a hundred years or more as a statement of defiance against the over-bearing nature of either state or family.

In the end it is important to remember that Puritanism was not only a spiritual matter, it was an attempt to establish a godly society on earth. In a hostile environment, there would always be pressure to separate and sometimes, as in England after the Restoration, exclusion would be enforced. But, in such circumstances, introversion and oppression are not the only possible defences. Stocker, for example, argues that in the post-Restoration period Puritans did not become more introverted in doctrinal matters; that is to say they continued to seek a godly society upon earth and to see earthly fortunes as a reflection of God's judgement of both individual and society (Stocker, 1992: 77; see also Morton, 1978). Whilst the political exuberance of the 1640s may have died, Stocker insists that 'political quietism is not equivalent to religious inversion'. Rather, she suggests that Puritans returned to their 'central myth . . . of a permanent spiritual "warfare" against the forces of darkness and oppression'. Puritans had always sought to live *in* the world, however much they may have wished not to be *of* it.

In the absence of clear evidence of changes in the actual behaviour of Puritan families, we are left with the problem of extrapolating from more literary forms of evidence. As we have seen, these have led writers like Morgan and Leverenz, both of whom have an acute ear for changes in Puritan language, to see in the later seventeenth century a growing introversion, an implosion almost, of the Puritan family. Sommerville, extrapolating more conventionally from political circumstances, comes to the same conclusion. Puritan parenting was perhaps always a high risk strategy; since the religious stakes were so high so, also, had to be the emotional risks. Lawrence Stone was right to put his finger upon the potent mixture of intense love and rigorous discipline but where he was wrong was seeing in rigour only rigidity and oppression. That was never the ideal and from little we can know, was not generally the practice either.

But other responses were possible. We have already noted how, late in the eighteenth century, the Taylor family found in their religion, not oppression, but a strong defence against an often hostile world. Long before the Taylors, however, a tinker turned itinerant preacher produced a text which put into the hands of parents a powerful weapon with which to fight the war against darkness and oppression. During the period of oppression of religious dissent after the

Restoration, the Baptist John Bunyan wrote and published *Pilgrim's Progress.* In his allegory of Christian's pilgrimage to the celestial city, Bunyan produced a panorama of the worldliness against which the Puritan tradition had always fought. Bunyan's characters, the obstacles to Christian's progress, are not merely to be resisted, fought with and conquered, but they are made fun of, mocked and ridiculed. *Pilgrim's Progress* was not written for children, but very rapidly it became a children's book, and for two and a half centuries it was adapted, edited, dramatised and remained a model and an inspiration for generations of writers for children (Bratton, 1981: Darton, 1982: Sommerville, 1992). Through the Sunday School Movement, it found its way into thousands of working-class as well as middle-class homes. The tradition it represents is one that demands action in the world, not a cowering away from it; it believes in human sinfulness, but finds escape from it in humour as well as in resistance; it presents evil in very human tangible forms and puts into the hands of the pilgrim tangible forms of defeating it. As Stocker suggests, whilst the journey of Christian is a solitary one in which he flees from his wife and children, the ultimate goal is familial and communal. In the second part of the story, Christiana and her children recapitulate his pilgrimage to reach the community of the celestial city (Stocker, 1992). Thus, at least in allegory, the conflict of family and individual finds some resolution.

Clearly, one can no more extrapolate from one book (however remarkable its impact) to judgements about the fate of Puritan parenting than one can from the political circumstances of the Restoration or from the changing language of Puritan writing. Nevertheless, it suggests a continuing vitality in the Puritan tradition in waging war against both the sinfulness of the self and of the world outside. One aspect of that war was the finding of a way to bring children up to develop and defend their own integrity, whilst keeping them not only involved in the world but prosperous and happy in it. For Puritans, of course, this was to be found only in a godly society, but their distinctive contribution was to seek the answer in reason *and* in feeling, in discipline *and* in love. Darton, perhaps, captures the problem this presents to us:

> That is a thing not to be forgotten in Puritanism – that its faith was an argument as well as an emotion. It becomes incomprehensible to us, perhaps even intolerable, when the argument asks too lofty, too perfect a standard in those to whom it is addressed. The

> impossibility of perfect goodness thus argued makes one forget the emotion that craves for it.
>
> (Darton, 1982: 65)

Romanticism did not, perhaps, forget the emotion that produced the fervency of Puritanism, but simply did not understand the implications for childhood to be derived from an utter conviction of the reality of original sin and of the need for salvation. That may have been due partly to the fragmentation and increasing voluntarism of religious belief, but it was also because the Enlightenment shaped new conceptions of childhood which were at odds with Augustinian theology and its doctrine of original sin. It is to these new conceptions that we must now turn.

Chapter 3

The child of the Enlightenment

The example of Locke and Rousseau

> My Dear Child: I am very well pleased with your last letter. The writing was very good, and the promise you made exceedingly fine. You must keep it, for an honest man never breaks his word. You engage to retain the instructions which I give you. That is sufficient, for though you do not properly comprehend them at present, age and reflection will, in time, make you understand them.
>
> Lord Chesterfield to his son at school, 1739.

> As for Hetty, She already knows so much of History, Geography, Astronomy & Natural Philosophy; that She now begins to study for her own sake, & does not so much require keeping to Hours as younger Children do; She has besides a sort of every-day-wit; a degree of Prudence, Discretion and common Sense, that I have seldom seen in a Girl even of twelve or thirteen Years old, which makes her a most comfortable Child; in spite of her bad Temper & cold heart; I really can consult her and often do – She is so *very* rational.
>
> Hester Thrale's diary, 1773.

The Enlightenment appears to have found little more favour with the Romantics than did Puritanism, and certainly few would now be prepared to view it as the philosopher Kant did as heralding the coming of age of human societies. To the Romantics and Victorians the 'age of reason' was a time of 'shallow and mechanical thinkers, overweeningly confident in abstract reason', who had no understanding of the 'imagination, feeling, the organic power of tradition and history, and the mysteries of the soul' (Porter, 1990: 2).

The twentieth century has been kinder than the nineteenth and generally more independent in its judgement than it has been of Puritanism, but here again late twentieth-century scholarship has tended to fragment the very notion of an Enlightenment, to destroy the generalities, so that the term itself increasingly needs justification for its use. Such disputes need not detain us long because there is no intention to describe a general Enlightenment view of childhood or child-rearing; rather the purpose of this chapter is to look in some detail at two figures whose contemplation of the business of educating children still commands attention at the end of the twentieth century, Locke and Rousseau. Of these, Locke requires a broad definition of the Enlightenment to be included, writing as he did in England towards the end of the seventeenth century. He has often been regarded as a founding father of the Enlightenment because ideas of his were so often taken and elaborated upon by eighteenth-century intellectuals. The eighteenth century may well have claimed him, but this is not without its problems in diverting attention away from his own intellectual and, especially, religious origins (Dunn, 1984; Spellman, 1988). Rousseau, on the other hand, belonged more clearly to the narrower intellectual school of the eighteenth-century French Enlightenment, but within that school, he was something of a rebel and an alienated voice.

It is too simplistic to oppose faith and reason and to see the Enlightenment as confronting the former with the latter. If there was an intellectual revolution, there is much to be said for locating it in the seventeenth-century when, in France, Descartes propounded reason as a distinctive way of thinking and as a skill to be learned and, in England, not only did the Civil War open traditional political thought to rationalist and sometimes extraordinarily radical ideas, but the Royal Society emerged to give shape and substance to Baconian ideas of a rational scientific method. Hill indeed claims of the seventeenth-century intellectual revolution that now 'it is difficult for us to conceive how men thought before it was made' (Hill, 1980: 163). But claiming revolutions in the history of ideas, and especially in relation to the tension between faith and reason, is always likely to overstate the case (Baumer, 1977). As we have seen, there was a strong rationalist strain in Puritanism, opposing the ritual and mysticism of Roman Catholicism, seeking an understanding of God's will through the exercise of the mind (Morgan, J., 1986; Stocker, 1992).

Nevertheless, the Enlightenment is still a descriptive term that conveys something significant about the development of the way in which human beings, and especially intellectuals amongst them, viewed the world in which they lived, and tried to shape it to their desires. As Porter puts it, Enlightenment thinkers 'were above all *critics*, aiming to put human intelligence to use as an engine for understanding human nature, for analysing man as a sociable being, and the natural environment in which he lived' (Porter, 1990: 3). It was a period, also, when a more sinister trend in the history of ideas emerged, not unassociated with reason; this is what Baumer refers to as a shift in emphasis from concepts of being to concepts of becoming; a shift of focus from the absolute to the relative, from the fixed state to the historical trend (Baumer, 1977: 20).

Amongst the many consequences of this gradual rupturing of theological and teleological certainties was a growing fascination with that changeable, changing and disordered period of human existence, childhood. Whilst the world remained fixed and certain, its purposes clear to God if not always comprehensible to humankind, then the child had to remain incomprehensible or be forced, willing or not, into what humankind imagined God's image of childhood to be. The doctrine of original sin had allowed conventional wisdom to give voice to this incomprehension in less than flattering ways. In 1688 the French satirist La Bruyere, for example, described children as, 'overbearing, supercilious, passionate, envious, inquisitive, egotistical, idle, fickle, timid, intemperate, liars and dissemblers' (La Bruyère, 1963: para. 50). A more sober writer, Pierre Bayle, was even more outspoken:

> In children nothing but evil inclinations are to be seen. Those who bring them up always find some vice to correct, and if the natural faults were not made good by threats, promises and good instruction, all children would become little villains and incapable of becoming anything of worth throughout their lives... our human nature is a spoiled and corrupted well, a soil accursed; for what are the first fruits which sooner or later it will bear – greed, pride, anger, avarice, jealousy, envy, lying, desire for luxury? It is not education which makes these seeds of evil grow; they are nearly all there before it and they burst into light because of the great obstacles with which education tries to oppose them. A child's mind is no better conditioned than its heart. They only judge things by the evidence of their senses; they examine nothing, they swallow errors without any mistrust, they believe blindly in the tales they are told.
>
> (quoted Labrousse, 1964: 78n)

Bayle was a Calvinist (a Protestant refugee in Holland when he was writing at the end of the seventeenth century) and might, therefore, be expected to have such pessimistic views of childhood. But there is more to Bayle than this, and his is amongst the most tragic visions of childhood. In the first place education does not eradicate or even counteract infant depravity, rather it serves to socialise and render infant passions respectable, turning greed into ambition, aggression into bravery and selfishness into self-interest. Furthermore, to the sins children are born with are added those learned from their parents. However, for those who adhere to the Fifth Commandment to 'Honour Your Father and Mother', these sins are learned through the exercise of a proper duty and in all innocence. The child, then, is caught between the charybdis of original sin and the scylla of duty to parents; growing up, honouring one's parents (themselves the products of original sin and of a corrupting education) leads to a deterioration, not improvement in the capacity to make rational judgements. Only adults who can effectively suppress the socialising effects of their childhood can hope to escape the cycle of depravity, and few succeed (Labrousse, 1964; 1983).

Bayle offered no systematic treatise upon childhood, but his scattered thoughts do disclose a tension which others were to explore more thoroughly. For Bayle the problem was not simply one of original sin, it was also one of education and socialisation. In the growing child it was impossible to distinguish between sinful behaviour which originated in the child's sinful nature and that which was the result of parental influence. Yet whilst responsibility for the former lay in the collective guilt of humankind, the latter was the result of children obeying God's commandment to honour their parents. The critical issue was the tendency of parental influence to damage the rational capacities of the child.

It is this shift of attention away from the effects of original sin, to the effects of socialisation – a growing environmentalism – which perhaps is the hallmark of the emerging Enlightenment. The fight to establish the innocence of the newborn child was begun in the late seventeenth century, but it was never an easy struggle and success has never been assured even in the late twentieth century. But, just as significantly, the Enlightenment implied a new, radical dimension to parental responsibility by suggesting a tension between the necessity of teaching and training the young child, and a desire to preserve the autonomy of the emerging adult. 'If', as Kessen observes, 'the nature of man is defined in the experience of the child, then man can mimic God and reconstruct himself. The history of the child for three hundred years has been the history of a dialogue on the conception of childhood as construction' (Kessen, 1965: 58). Kessen undoubtedly captures something of the spirit that was abroad in the Enlightenment, but he over-simplifies the problem. Intellectually, if not emotionally, the Puritan father may have found it easier to play God to his children, since the goal of Puritan parenting was not the child's autonomy. The hypothetical parents and tutors which emerge in the writings of Locke and Rousseau have to tread a fine line between constructing children in their own image and recognising the integrity of each individual child. Subsequent judges of both Locke and Rousseau have been far from convinced that they got the balance right.

JOHN LOCKE

> Mens Happiness or Misery is most part of their own making. He, whose Mind directs not wisely, will never take the right Way...
>
> of all the men we meet with, Nine Parts of ten are what they are, Good or Evil, useful or not, by their Education.
>
> I imagine the Minds of Children as easily turned this or that way, as Water it self...
>
> (Locke *Some Thoughts Concerning Education*: para. 1–2)

These opening remarks from Locke's *Some Thoughts Concerning Education* appear to contain a contradiction. On the one hand Locke is saying that people are responsible for their own lives, but on the other he stresses the extent to which they are determined by their education. On the one hand the 'Mind' must direct the individual to behave appropriately; on the other the 'Mind' of the child is as easily directed as water. There is a sense in which Locke here is expressing the same dilemma that haunted Bayle: that, as adults we have to take responsibility for our actions, but already our mind has been shaped, for good or bad, by forces which acted upon us in the weakness of our childhood.

Locke's *Some Thoughts Concerning Education* constitutes an attempt to describe in detailed, practical ways an upbringing and an education which will fit the child for the adult world. The question we need to ask, therefore, is whether Locke's proposals succeed in preparing the child for adult life without debilitating and corrupting the mind in the way Bayle suggests. What kind of upbringing does he propose and what is the role of parents and teachers in it? It will be apparent, when we turn to Rousseau, that he, too, was preoccupied with the same dilemma.

There are some real difficulties in gauging the significance of *Some*

Thoughts that need to be stated at the outset. At the most general level there is the relationship of Locke to those followers who claimed him as an environmentalist, who believed in the power of education and played down the influence of human nature. Did he really believe in the perfectibility of humankind (Passmore, 1970)? As Spellman has noted, if this were Locke's position, it would indeed have been radical for the late seventeenth century, but, in practice, Locke's thought is much more constrained by his time and the concept of an inborn, inbred human nature is very much part of it. It is more important to recognise that, whatever a strict reading of the text may indicate, unspoken assumptions are just as important. These assumptions, says Spellman, were 'never plainly articulated because they were a part of the common intellectual inheritance of the late seventeenth century, the very warp and woof of a long-standing world view' (Spellman, 1988: 206). In Lovejoy's terms it is important to play as much attention to the 'metaphysical pathos' that surrounds a debate as to the cerebral arguments themselves (Lovejoy, 1936). There are occasions when one can sense the tension between a principle and a reality, and between a sense of what is and what should be. Such detailed instances merit as much attention as the grand generalisations but they much less often receive it.

A second problem lies in this very specific and practical orientation of *Some Thoughts*. There is a difficulty in knowing to what extent proper appreciation is really dependent upon an understanding of Locke's other writings. It was, after all, not intended as a systematic treatise, but was rather the revision of letters sent to a friend who had asked for advice about bringing up his son (Yolton, 1989). And, as advice addressed to the parents of one who was to be a gentleman with all that that entailed, what relevance has it as a general treatise on education? It would be surprising, however, if one of Locke's great intellectual imagination did not attempt to see a broader pattern behind the practical advice he offered, and though the social range of the application of his advice was undoubtedly limited, it certainly goes beyond the limits of the courtesy book upon which it was, to some degree, modelled.

In any case there is no escaping the fact that we always read such a text in two ways. First we read in search of the meaning and significance which belongs to its own time which we need to discover if we are fully to understand its significance. But second we inevitably read against our experience of the present in a search for what might be relevant, curious, sometimes funny, sometimes disturbing for us.

Where we are most likely to go wrong is if we assume we can do one thing without the other. We need also to bear in mind that the status of such a text changes radically through time. For us it never can be, in any simple sense, a work of practical advice on education, but for generations of the upper classes in the eighteenth century it certainly was. Lawrence Stone identifies it as one of the 'key instruments' in the propagation of bourgeois domestic thought in the eighteenth century, going through some twenty-five editions in the century after its first appearance in 1693 (Stone, 1979: 175, 279).

What then are the principles which underlie Locke's approach to education? His world view is predominantly religious, tolerant and unspecific in the details of belief, but committed to the inescapable duty to search for and follow the law of nature which is the law of God. The essential characteristic of human beings is that they have the ability to act according to reason and in this lies their freedom. This leads to an eclectic theology combining a Calvinist sense of duty with an underlying rationalism (Parry, 1978: 27; Dunn, 1984). It has also lead to disputes about Locke's view of original sin. Some see in Locke the legacy of his own Puritan childhood – his father was a captain in the parliamentary army – and of the Protestant tradition in general (Dunn, 1984; Yolton, 1989; Spellman, 1988); whilst others claim to find an almost complete rejection of all forms of the theological doctrine of original sin (Schouls, 1992). Detailed intertextual reading of Locke's whole output might support Schouls, but perhaps writers like Dunn sense the weight of tradition and feeling, the 'metaphysical pathos', more clearly. Undoubtedly he believed children had natural inclinations, which would lead them away from the path of virtue. Children love liberty, he notes, and for that reason should not be unduly restrained, but he continues

> I now tell you, they love something more; and that is *Dominion*: And this is the first Original of most vicious Habits, that are ordinary and natural. This Love of *Power* and Dominion shews itself very early.
>
> (*Some Thoughts*: para. 103)

However, if we look at just one example, his discussion of children inflicting pain upon animals, it illustrates a much more ambiguous attitude. Of one thing Locke is sure: exposure to violence and the practising of violence accustom the child to its acceptance. This applies not only to the killing and tormenting of animals but also to the glorification of conquerors 'who for the most part are but the great Butchers of Mankind' (ibid.: para. 116). Locke talks with the approval of a mother who encouraged her daughters to keep pets so that they learned to take responsibility for them. Nevertheless, Locke believes there is a strain of cruelty in children, a 'delight they take in *doing of Mischief*, whereby I mean spoiling of anything to no purpose; but more especially the Pleasure they take to put anything in Pain that is capable of it' (ibid.: para. 116). As Schouls suggests, Locke's 'spoiling of anything to no purpose' is 'not a bad generic definition of sin' (1992: 199) and hence, perhaps, evidence of a belief in the inherent evil in the child. But Locke draws back from the brink, saying that he cannot persuade himself that this tendency to cruelty in children,

> be other than a foreign and introduced Disposition, an habit borrowed from Custom and Conversation. People teach Children to strike, and laugh, when they hurt, or see harm come to others.
> (*Some Thoughts*: para. 116)

Locke's environmentalist leanings are rarely so clearly expressed. The purpose of education is to bring the child to virtue, which in practice, as the details of *Some Thoughts* make clear, is to an achievement of rational moral behaviour in the community of humankind; learning and accomplishments fall some way behind in importance (Yolton, 1989). It is undoubtedly a more secular vision of godly behaviour than the Puritan saints would have recognised. Nevertheless, for Locke, the business of education was not finished until 'the young Man had a true relish of... [virtue], and placed his Strength, his Glory, and his Pleasure in it' (*Some Thoughts*: para. 70). Few children, however, naturally seek virtue, and the purpose of education is to correct the different inclinations and biases of each child so that vice is cured and virtue attained (ibid.: para. 139).

The great difference between Locke and the majority of Puritan writers lies in his attitude to religious belief. Locke's tolerance over matters of belief releases so many of the tensions that surrounded Puritanism. The transition from godliness to virtue is a subtle but significant one. What it achieves is a shift from an always incipient tendency to introversion (to prayer, to constant self-examination and remorse) to a much more extrovert definition of virtue as the proper conduct of one human being in the company of others. In this, of course, he is not particularly innovative, rather he follows an approach to education which can be found in the humanist tradition, and which always played down the significance of original sin

(Bantock, 1980). Nevertheless the religious ambience of Locke is strong, but it is a religion concerned with ethics rather than belief.

What then of Locke's method of education? It is worth recalling that within the broad Puritan tradition, the preparationist case was always strong. Puritan parents were unwilling to rely upon the grace of God or the rituals and ceremonies of churches in the upbringing of their children; hence the conflict between the simple pleasures that young children brought to parents (with the consequent temptation to indulge them), and the terror of eternal damnation which lead to a fearfulness about enjoying these same pleasures (Morgan, 1986). As with earlier writers of clear Puritan persuasion, Locke is concerned to establish parental authority early, or to be more precise, to establish the authority of *reason* through the parent; both parent and child are to be constrained by reason.

> The great Mistake I have observed in People's breeding their Children has been, that this has not been taken care enough of in *due season*; That the mind has not been made obedient to Discipline and pliant to Reason, when at first it was most tender, most easy to be bowed. Parents, being wisely ordain'd by Nature to love their Children, are very apt, if Reason watch not that natural Affection very warily, are apt, I say, to let it run into fondness. They love their little ones, and 'tis their Duty: But they often, with them, cherish their Faults too. They must not be crossed, forsooth: they must be permitted to have their Wills in all things: and they being in their Infancies not capable of great Vices, their Parents think they may safely indulge their little irregularities, and make themselves Sport with that pretty perverseness, which, they think, well enough becomes that innocent Age.
>
> (*Some Thoughts*: para. 34)

Here Locke observes the tension between love and discipline that so much exercised Puritan thought about child-rearing; it is, however, the emphasis upon reason which marks the difference. Even so, Locke insists that children should learn self-denial 'even in their cradles' and that their will should be obedient to that of their parents' from as early an age as possible. They should learn to look upon them as 'their Lords, their Absolute Governors' with fear and awe (ibid.: paras 39–41). Locke expresses particular concern about the consequences of following indulgence and familiarity in infancy with severity and distance in later years, since this will not lead to the respect and love that parents should hope to receive from their grown-up children.

That will only come when children, themselves, have grown to appreciate the force of reason which was exercised on their behalf in infancy.

Locke modifies this apparently severe regime by frequently stressing the necessity that parents ask no more of children than their capacities can manage. Children are creatures who 'must play, and have Play-things' (ibid.: para. 39). Even their faults are to be overlooked upon occasion:

> For, All their innocent Folly, Playing, and *Childish Actions*, are to be left perfectly free and *unrestrained*, as far as they can consist with the Respect due to those that are present; and that with the greatest Allowance. If these Faults of their Age, rather than of the Children themselves, were, as they should be, left only to Time and Imitation, and riper Years to cure, Children would escape a great deal of misapplied and useless Correction.
>
> (ibid.: para. 63)

However rigorous the discipline, it must not produce 'dejected minds' and 'low spirits' (ibid.: para. 46), and Locke's discussion of corporal punishment mirrors very closely that of his Puritan predecessors in seeing it as a sign of failure on the part of parents, to be used only as a last resort. Learning should be fun, like play, and the 'true Secret of Education' is to find the balance between the need to restrain and the need to encourage the 'Child's Spirit, easy and free'.

Understanding the child's nature and taking account of its development is central to Locke's approach to education. But what is this nature? In what way does the child approach the business of learning? Locke's metaphor of the infant mind as white paper is perhaps his best known image but also the most confusing. It has been taken to imply passivity on the part of the child and equality between human beings, neither of which Locke intended; his child is very active in absorbing and understanding what it sees, hears and feels, and though Locke rates the natural abilities of humankind very highly, he stresses the different temperaments and inclinations which are individual to each child (Yolton, 1985: 134; 1989: 38). Some recent commentators have stressed the notion of vulnerability that is inherent in the image, and if one considers the general tone of Locke's comments about children, not only in *Some Thoughts*, but also in *An Essay Concerning Human Understanding* where the metaphor first appears, then this general meaning gains significance (Neill, 1991: Schouls, 1992).

Locke is fearful of the impact that the world makes upon the growing child, about the prejudices and general misinformation that are likely to emanate from nurses and servants at home and from fellow pupils at school. 'We are a sort of Camelions, that still take a Tincture from things near us', he says (*Some Thoughts*: para. 68). Locke's dislike of schools is well known. However, his objection is not to the teachers but to the peer-group:

> how any one's being put into a mixed Herd of unruly boys, and there learning to wrangle at Trap, or rook at Span-farthing, fits him [the child] for civil Conversation, or Business, I do not see. And what Qualities are ordinarily to be got from such a Troop of Play-fellows as Schools usually assemble together from Parents of all kinds, that a Father should so much covet, is hard to define.
>
> (ibid.: para. 70)

Locke's concern with vulnerability even extends to some degree to the children of the poor for whom he wished to provide the kind of education that their parents could not provide, parents that Locke thought 'offended' in 'not opening their children's minds' (quoted Schouls, 1992: 180). This suggests more than the narrow vocationalism usually attributed to Locke's view of education for the masses.

'Vulnerability', notes Schouls, 'is one side of the coin. The other side is that of opportunity' (Schouls, 1992: 191). The opportunity is to be free of the constraints of prejudice inflicted upon the child during its years of intellectual dependence and to test tradition and custom against reason. The opportunity comes through the exercise of reason and hence the critical task of education is to develop reason within the growing child.

> He that is not used to submit his Will to the Reason of others, *when* he is *young*, will scarce harken or submit to his own Reason, when he is of an Age to make use of it.
>
> (*Some Thoughts*: para. 36)

The apparent conflict between Locke's insistence upon the development of good habits in the development of virtue, and the need to develop the exercise of reason unshackled by the weight of custom is resolved (intellectually at least) by Locke's insistence that the habits to be taught are those of method, not of belief or behaviour – in other words, children are to be taught the habit of rational thought (Neill, 1991; Schouls, 1992). Locke's technique is simplicity itself. Treat children as if they *are* rational; accord to rational behaviour esteem and to irrational behaviour disgrace. Thus, the innate tendency of all human beings to seek pleasure and avoid pain will lead them towards rational behaviour.

> It will perhaps be wondered at that I mention *Reasoning* with Children: And yet I cannot but think that the true Way of Dealing with them. They understand it as early as they do Language: and, if I mistake not, they love to be treated as Rational Creatures sooner than is imagined. 'Tis a Pride should be cherished in them, and, as much as can be, made the great Instrument to turn them by.
>
> (*Some Thoughts*: para. 81)

Thus Locke attempts to break out of the dilemma posed so dramatically by Bayle by insisting upon an education which does not instill habitual patterns of behaviour and belief, but provides the child with the rational tools to take responsibility for their own conduct. It is a programme which often demonstrates an intuitive insight into and sensitivity for the needs and nature of children, but very little understanding of the frailties of parents. More generally, there is a belief in the infallibility of reason which, as Schouls intimates, suggests a belief which is born of enthusiasm rather than evidence. Locke shared with many in the late seventeenth century a dislike of religious enthusiasm (it was a criticism levelled against the heirs of the Puritan tradition), but he himself was guilty of a similar enthusiasm, not for religion but for reason itself (Schouls, 1992: 231).

If, for the Puritans, the role of the parent was to represent God to the child, for Locke, their role was to represent reason until the child's own capacities were able to make independent judgements. For the Puritans, the wealth and richness of the imagery which surrounded God as parent demanded both empathy with the child in the form of the loving, nurturing mother, and distance in the shape of the governing father. Locke softens the role of father and he makes little gender distinction when referring to either parents or children (Leites, 1981: 101). He demands a much more specific empathy with the nature of the individual child, its inclinations and pattern of development, but perhaps he requires less empathy with the child's emotional state. As Leites complains, Locke denies to the growing child the legitimacy of enthusiasm and ecstasy (Leites, 1981: 110). The ecstasy of love, which is never far below the surface of Puritan fervency, seems to find little place in Locke's education.

Parental authority in Locke

It is not surprising that, in the political theory of Locke's *Two Treatises of Government*, family relationships should find a mention, not merely as a metaphor for civil relationships in general, but as something worth consideration in their own right. Indeed, it is almost inconceivable that any seventeenth-century political debate should not make some reference, however conventional, to authority within family relationships. In his discussions, Locke is much concerned to refute the doctrine of patriarchal sovereignty. In particular, he sets out to destroy the argument of one, Sir Robert Filmer, whose tract *Patriarcha* had achieved some fame in the years leading up to the revolution of 1688.

Filmer had rested his case for royal absolutism squarely upon the analogy of the natural authority of a father over his child. 'The argument from fatherhood', says Schochet, 'was not just one of several supports for monarchy; it was the bedrock itself' (Schochet, 1975: 139). Indeed the fact of the child's dependence upon his parents was so obvious that it could be used as a basis for arguing that since children clearly had no *de facto* freedom or equality as infants, there could be no basis for arguing that human beings, in general, were either free or equal. Filmer is clear and succinct on this issue: 'Every man that is born is so far from being free, that by his very birth he becomes a subject of him that begets him'(quoted ibid.: 125). Indeed as Archbishop Tenison put it at the end of the century, to tell people they were born free and equal was 'to put some such cheat upon the World, as Nurses are wont, in sport, to put upon unwary Children, when they tell them, they started out of the Parsleybed' (quoted ibid.: 184). Not only was it a cheat to tell people they were free, but the implications of such a proposition were absurd since, as Filmer argued, to allow everybody to have a voice in the establishment of government would result, because of numerical superiority, in giving 'the children the government over their parents' (quoted ibid.: 125).

Whilst the obvious weakness of the patriarchalist argument lay in the assumption that the relationship of father to child was necessarily the model for government, the fact that they emphasised the familial relationship so strongly presented contractualist writers such as Locke with something of a problem. The problem lay not so much in political theory, perhaps, as in the need to present their own view of family relationships. Seventeenth-century political debates were replete with references to family relationships and, in particular, to the father–child relationship. Even though the issue under debate was about the nature of political authority, it was impossible to discuss this without commenting upon the nature of family authority. Thus discussing childhood as a symbol of political subservience involved Locke in stating his own views as to the real nature of childhood dependence.

Hobbes, with characteristically ruthless logic, had rejected procreation as a justification for authority and attributed childhood dependence simply to the power first of all of the mother, to succour or kill her infant, and then to that of the father who had a similar power of life and death over both mother and child. The child was deemed to have given its 'consent' to the father's absolute authority out of gratitude for having saved its life when in a state of utter dependence. But for most writers such a rejection of the naturalness of paternal authority was too great a break with tradition. Some referred to the particular quality of the relationship between parent and child, to its gentleness and benevolence, distinguishing it from the harsher, more rigorous relationships of the adult world. Others, such as Tyrrell (a friend of Locke's), stressed the duty of parents to see to the upbringing of their children. Tyrrell saw parents as acting as trustees for their children during their period of nonage. Filmer, on the other hand, had denied that such a conception existed in nature: either a child was born free or human beings were never free. But Tyrrell insisted,

> There really is an Age of Nonage in nature . . . in which though the child be indeed free, yet (by reason of his own want of strength and discretion) is obliged to submit himself to his Parents' judgment in all things conducing to that end.
>
> (quoted ibid.: 149)

It is this approach, too, that Locke adopts. His problem is clear enough; he must deny the relevance of familial power to the question of political authority, whilst preserving the natural relationships of the family itself. In the *Two Treatises* Locke distinguishes three sorts of power: paternal, political and despotic. What distinguishes these three is their effect upon an individual's property, by which Locke means, not only property in goods, but the 'property' of an individual as a person, their individual abilities and characteristics. Under despotic power, people have no control over their property, whilst under political power, in Locke's definition, they do. The third type of power is paternal power, and Locke makes it clear that he does not believe this to be an absolute power, as conceived by either Filmer or Hobbes. In the *Second Treatise* he says,

> It is true, the paternal is a natural government, but not at all extending itself to the ends and jurisdictions of that which is political. The power of the father doth not reach at all to the property of the child, which is only in his own disposing.
>
> (Book 2: para. 170)

In abstract terms, the child's own self (its property) is its own, and in that sense the child can be born free and equal. Nevertheless, Locke acknowledges the natural government of the parent (and he includes the mother in that government), and consequently has to make childhood a special state where the theoretical freedom is accepted but the requirements of the child's dependent state are understood. Locke stresses the role of parents in carrying out the duty to their offspring imposed by God, and talks of 'the affection and tenderness God hath planted in the breasts of parents', and of their 'suitable inclinations of tenderness and concern' (ibid.: para. 170, 63; see also Book 1: para. 97).

To counter Filmer, Locke gives special attention to the significance of the Fifth Commandment. In Book 1 of the *Two Treatises* he rejects the idea that familial power can have implications for political power, basically on the grounds that it is a *non sequitur*. In Book 2 he devotes a whole chapter to the nature of paternal power, drawing together his thoughts upon the relationship of the child to the adult (Book 2: Chapter 6). Here he provides a particularly clear and full exposition of his views on the child–adult relationship in which his broader conception of human nature is modified to take account of the special status of childhood. Thus on equality, he says,

> Children . . . are not born in this full state of equality, though they are born to it. Their parents have a sort of rule and jurisdiction over them when they come into the world, and for some time after, but it is but a temporary one.
>
> (ibid.: para. 55)

The government of parents is to be based upon reason, supplying the understanding which the child lacks, but that reason is to be exercised for the child's own freedom:

> Thus, we are born free as we are born rational: not that we have actually the exercise of either: age that brings one, brings with it the

> other too. And thus we see how natural freedom and subjugation to parents may consist together, and both are founded on the same principle. A child is free by his father's title, by his father's understanding which is to govern him till he hath it of his own.
>
> (ibid.: para. 61)

The role of parents is therefore clear, it

> arises from that duty which is incumbent on them, to take care of their offspring during the imperfect state of childhood. To inform the mind, and govern the actions of their yet ignorant nonage till reason shall take its path and ease them of that trouble, is what the children want, and the parents are bound to.
>
> (ibid.: para. 58)

God's injunction in the Fifth Commandment has now a power and meaning which is mostly lacking in the protestations of Locke's patriarchalist opponents:

> He has laid on the children a perpetual obligation of honouring their parents, which, containing in it an inward esteem and reverence to be shown by all outward expressions, ties up the child from anything that may ever injure or affront, disturb or endanger the happiness or life of those from whom he received his, and engages him in all actions of defence, relief, assistance, and comfort of those by whose means he entered into being and has been made capable of any enjoyments of life. From this obligation no state, no freedom, can absolve children.
>
> (ibid.: para. 66)

Locke's conception of childhood

What makes Locke important in any discussion of childhood is that he was driven to face the problems of childhood through his basic concerns with the nature of the human mind and with the proper relationships that ought to exist between adults in civil society. As Archard says, 'Locke exemplifies a philosophical tradition of understanding children in a mixture of epistemological, educational and political terms' (Archard, 1993: 10). As Archard demonstrates, Locke is not without his problems, but he did establish two things. First, that the child is of the same nature as the adult, intellectually, socially and politically; second that the child needs to be brought up within some special social space, protected by parents and teachers. In this space, the adult has to express for the child those qualities of freedom and reason which are as yet only potentialities in childhood's 'imperfect state'. Thus a close bond is established between adult and child in that the former must be the adult in the child before the latter can assume responsibility for himself.

However, this relationship is held in balance by the recognition of an overriding duty to live according to God's law of nature. In terms of the concepts of being and becoming, Locke illustrates well the emerging conflict. On the one had there is an emphasis upon method in learning rather substance, upon the way the mind must reflect upon sensations to form ideas, and his insistence that authority be tested by individual reason; all of which suggests a move towards relativity and subjectivism (Bantock, 1980). These propositions come from the intellect. On the other hand, there is a profound belief in the fixed order of God's creation, in humankind's duty, and in the need to find certainty of knowledge and purpose by restricting the ambitions of the mind. Here is the underlying metaphysical pathos; an affection for an ordered, controlled life with a clear destiny. Nowhere does this conflict come out more clearly than in Locke's discussion of childhood. What the intellect will admit as being correct for the adult, or for humankind in general, the underlying emotion cannot accept for children. This is made most evident in *Some Thoughts*, where he makes Learning subservient to Virtue, Wisdom and Breeding in his educational aims. For Virtue, a knowledge of God is essential, but that knowledge should involve no metaphysical speculation; rather an uncritical acceptance of His existence and His law. Similarly, Wisdom is not to be taught, but is a matter of acquiring the right habits, as is Breeding. Learning is placed last, and is to consist of a general introduction to knowledge, rather than an attempt to gain the mastery of a subject that might lead to premature speculation (*Some Thoughts*: para. 136). As Bantock says,

> There are, then, whole areas of human behaviour which must be 'implanted', 'fashioned', 'worked into', made habitual, derived from 'imitation', acquired without that questioning that Locke seems to consider the essential function of the understanding. . . . 'Autonomy' is to be confined to the area of understanding – it is not appropriate to certain vital areas of conduct.
>
> (Bantock, 1980: 240)

In shaping both the mentality and politics of liberal societies, Locke exhibits a tendency with respect to childhood which remains, even in the twentieth century, significant. First, and most strikingly, he draws a sharp distinction between the contractual relationships of adults one to another, and the natural familial relationships that exist between parent and child. In establishing the political criteria for relationships between human beings in general, he specifically and categorically excludes children from those relationships. Within liberal society, childhood must be regarded as a special case. Second, though more equivocally, in edging towards a conception of humankind as intellectually self-conscious, critical and autonomous, Locke must of necessity emphasise the definition of the child as incomplete, inadequate and 'imperfect'. Having defined the dependence of the child in terms of the autonomy of the adult, Locke leaves subsequent generations, lacking his powerful theology of the family, intellectually searching for new ways of rationalising dependency and seeking new justifications for parental authority.

JEAN-JACQUES ROUSSEAU

The problem for the Enlightenment is well described by Bantock. In turning to a secular view of nature as the basis of order in civilisation, they followed an empirical scientific tradition developed in the previous century, but they tried also to assimilate humankind into this empiricist world, searching for similar laws of nature to govern their conduct. They confused, as it were, ethical and factual truth, and clinging to a teleological view of humankind sought a sense of moral purpose in scientific laws (Bantock, 1980: 255). Not surprisingly, they often found themselves confused. Hence the anxious bemusement of Diderot:

> O God, I do not know if you exist. . . . I ask nothing in this world, for the course of events is determined by its own necessity if you do NOT exist, or by your decree if you DO. . . . Here I stand, as I am, a necessarily organised part of eternal matter or perhaps your own creation.
>
> (quoted in Hampson, 1968: 96)

The legacy of Locke, then, proved to be difficult. As Spellman has argued, the eighteenth century tended to play down the religious context and feeling that pervades Locke's work, and to use his writing as the basis of an increasingly environmentalist position on education especially (Spellman, 1988: 2).

Rousseau was, however, singularly unimpressed with the products of social engineering that he saw around him; he saw not progress but corruption. Undoubtedly part of the Enlightenment, but never fully belonging, this deeply alienated man sought to reassess the relationship between humankind and the natural world. Faced with what he believed to be a profoundly corrupt society, Rousseau strove to re-establish the integrity of human nature and through this to forge a new society. In his *Discourse on the Origins of Inequality*, written in the middle of the eighteenth century, Rousseau describes the fall of humankind in terms of the corrupting effects of society as it developed from primitive innocence to sophisticated perversion (Rousseau, 1973). Thus, as Broome so aptly put it, Rousseau 'socialises sin . . . – transferring the responsibility and the burden of guilt from men as individuals to men collectively' (Broome, 1963: 17). A few years later in the *Emile*, Rousseau opened with a similar theme:

> Everything is good as it leaves the hands of the Author of things; everything degenerates in the hands of man. He forces one soil to nourish the products of another, one tree to bear the fruit of another. He mixes and confuses the climates, the elements, the seasons. He mutilates his dog, his horse, his slave. He turns everything upside down; he disfigures everything: he loves deformity, monsters. He wants nothing as nature made it, not even man; for him, man must be trained like a school horse; man must be fashioned in keeping with his fancy like a tree in his garden.
>
> (*Emile*: 37)

Thus human reason, in seeking to control nature, has achieved only distortion. For Rousseau, reason should rather emerge from nature, become nature 'turned reflective in moral wisdom' (Lloyd, 1984: 58).

By blaming society for corruption, Rousseau elevates childhood to a special place of innocence. Whilst conventionally the child was regarded, for good or bad, as free from the trappings and customs of adult society, Rousseau turns this aspect of childhood into a central part of his programme for social renewal. Infant innocence becomes something to be preserved, the tabula rasa image is subtly changed from neutrality to something with more positive, more creative potential.

It would be quite wrong, however, to think that the natural state of childhood represents a state of perfection. Again in the *Discourse on the Origins of Inequality*, Rousseau explains what he means by a state of nature. From a contemplation of 'the first and most simple operations of the human soul', Rousseau believes he can identify 'two principles prior to reason'. Of these two principles the first makes human beings deeply interested in their own welfare and preservation, but the other excites 'a natural repugnance at seeing any other sensible being, and particularly any of our own species, suffer pain and death' (Rousseau, 1973: 40). These notions of self-love (*amour de soi*) and pity are the basic motivations of humankind. In their original state, natural human beings are free, but free only because they live in isolation; Rousseau specifically avoids including sociability amongst the natural human characteristics. Humans are to be distinguished from the rest of the animal world, however, because of their ability to choose, though this difference has a moral and metaphysical quality about it rather than an intellectual one. He has also one further characteristic which places human beings apart in nature: this is their potential for perfection or, as Rousseau puts it, a 'faculty for self-improvement, which, by the help of circumstances, gradually develops all the rest of our facilities, and is inherent in the species as in the individual' (Rousseau, 1973: 54).

In this state of nature we live a life of innocence and happiness without society, but having a capacity for perfectibility and for virtue which places us apart from the animal world. The transition from nature to society was bound to change human beings but they have changed for the worse when they might have changed for the better. *Amour de soi* is a natural instinct and one which, if it had been 'directed in man by reason and modified by pity', could have produced 'humanity and virtue' (quoted Charvet, 1974: 12). But instead another form of self-love developed which Rousseau terms *amour propre*. This is entirely the product of society and consists of a self-evaluation which is dependent upon what other people think. Thus social beings come to live outside themselves, knowing how to live only through the opinion and judgement of others, their consciousness of their own existence coming only through relationships with others (Rousseau, 1973).

The project of *Emile* is to try to preserve the integrity of the growing child as it passes from innocence to virtue. The *Emile* is a curious work for the modern reader, half philosophical treatise, but increasingly towards the end a novel; occasionally a child-rearing manual, but seldom only that. It traces the infancy, childhood, adolescence and early manhood of Emile and especially his upbringing and education under the guidance of his infinitely wise Tutor. It also introduces Sophie, destined to become Emile's wife, and discourses upon her education and upon the role of women generally. However, central to

Rousseau's aim in *Emile* is to establish the nature of childhood itself and to explore the process of growing up and entering into social relationships.

In the Preface, Rousseau makes it quite clear that, in his view, there has been a tendency to look in the wrong direction:

> Childhood is unknown. Starting from the false idea one has of it, the farther one goes, the more one loses one's way. The wisest men concentrate on what it is important for men to know without considering what children are in a condition to learn. They are always seeking the man in the child without thinking of what he is before being a man.
>
> (*Emile*: 34)

It is possible to exaggerate the differences between Locke and Rousseau, but there is a sense in which Rousseau does set out to contradict one of Locke's central premises. Whilst Locke is prepared to acknowledge childhood capacities and inclinations, it is true, as Rousseau complains, that he is looking for the 'man' in the child and seeking, in particular, to develop the capacity for reason as soon as possible. For Rousseau, this position is reversed; childhood must be seen in its own terms as a natural state with its own natural development, not to be contradicted or interfered with by the adult, however much they may believe they are acting in the best long-term interests of the child. As Masters points out, Rousseau has a profound sense of history: it is not possible to know where a person will end, but it is possible to know where they start (Masters, 1968: 5). The present which is known should not be sacrificed to an unknown and unknowable future.

The aim of Rousseau's education of the young Emile is to allow him to learn from nature. To this end, it is critical that Emile learns nothing from the authority of an elder, but only from direct experience of the natural world. This 'negative education', frequently mocked as a wasteful exercise in reinventing the wheel, is less an end in itself, rather it expresses a concern that Emile should not be subject to the questionable wisdom of those older than himself. In so far as Locke strove to educate the child in *method* rather than in knowledge, both share a distrust of feeding the child with human knowledge when they lack the developed critical faculties to assess its worth. Thus, books are, with the notable exception of Defoe's *Robinson Crusoe*, banned by Rousseau and learning is to take place by direct discoveries made through experimentation with the physical environment. Locke would probably not have disagreed too much with the following sentiments:

> Let us transform our sensations into ideas but not leap all of a sudden from objects of sense to intellectual objects. It is by way of the former that we ought to get to the latter. In the first operations of the mind let the senses always be its guides. No book other than the world, no instruction other than the facts. The child who reads does not think, he only reads; he is not informing himself, he learns words.
>
> (*Emile*: 168)

Rousseau is concerned to avoid precocity and to ensure that, on the part of the adult, no premature judgements are made about the child's abilities and temperament; childhood, he warns, is 'reason's sleep' (ibid.: 107). In a direct criticism of Locke, he complains of children whose mentors attempt to reason with them.

> To reason with children was Locke's great maxim. It is the one most in vogue today. Its success, however, does not appear to me such as to establish its reputation: and, as for me, I see nothing more stupid than these children who have been reasoned with so much.
>
> (ibid.: 89)

Perhaps the most important break with Locke, however, comes in their respective attitudes to dependence and authority. Locke insisted on the dependence of the child upon the authority of the adult until the capacity for independent rational thought was gained; only through adult control of the will of the young child could virtue be achieved. Underlying the whole of Rousseau's discussion of the pre-adolescent phase of education, however, is the belief that the child should remain dependent upon things, rather than people, because things belong to nature and cannot corrupt, but people belong to society and are thereby corrupted. Emile must never act from obedience, but from necessity, demands Rousseau,

> Thus the words *obey* and *command* will be proscribed from his lexicon, and even more so *duty* and *obligation*. But *strength, necessity, impotence*, and *constraint* should play a great role in it. Before the age of reason one cannot have any idea of moral beings or of social relations. Hence so far as possible words which express them must be avoided.
>
> (ibid.: 89)

The natural domination of the adult over the child is one of force not reason; Emile should never be manipulated.

> Command him nothing, whatever in the world it might be, absolutely nothing. Do not even allow him to imagine that you might pretend to have any authority over him. Let him know only that he is weak and you are strong, that by his condition and yours he is necessarily at your mercy. Let him know it, learn it, feel it. Let his haughty head at an early date feel the harsh yoke which nature imposes upon man, the heavy yoke of necessity under which every finite thing must bend.
>
> (ibid.: 91)

In an echo of Bayle's tragic vision, he continues,

> It is quite strange that since people first became involved with raising children, no instrument for guiding them has been imagined other than emulation, jealousy, envy, vanity, avidity, and vile fear.
>
> (ibid.: 91)

Yet, change the tone of the language only slightly and what Rousseau so vehemently condemns are in fact the very instruments of control ('vile fear' apart) that Locke advocated as infinitely preferable to corporal punishment; not of course that Rousseau was advocating the latter.

With the development of abstract reasoning at about the age of 15 comes an even greater change, not merely cognitive but emotional:

> We are . . . born twice: once to exist, and once to live; once for our species and once for our sex. . . . As the roaring of the sea precedes a tempest from far away, this stormy revolution is proclaimed by the murmur of the nascent passions. . . . It is now that man is truly born to life and now that nothing human is foreign to him.
>
> (ibid.: 211)

It is only during adolescence that Emile is allowed to learn about his fellow human beings and about the moral world, not through direct experience, which Rousseau admits would be too dangerous, but by secondary means. This is now possible because Emile, having learned so far only through experience and not through authorities, is self-possessed enough to deal with the opinions of others. What is critical about adolescence, however, is the advent of the passions, particularly sexual feelings; these have to be channelled and harmonised, not repressed, so that Emile may develop into a fully human being. Having entered, as it were, into possession of himself, Emile is now ready to cease to be a child, says Rousseau. The task is to make the adolescent loving and tender hearted, to perfect reason through feeling (Rusk, 1979: 123).

In this most critical stage of education, in the transition from self-possessed child to social being, reason is ultimately to be seen as the servant of the most basic and natural instincts. Self-love (*amour de soi*), in itself naturally good, is to be transformed through pity into virtue. Emile must begin by relating his own suffering to that of others:

> At sixteen the adolescent knows what it is to suffer for he has himself suffered. But he hardly knows that other beings suffer too. To see it without feeling it is not to know it . . . the child, not imagining what others feel, knows only his own ills. But when the first development of his senses lights the fire of imagination, he begins to feel himself in his fellows, to be moved by their complaints and to suffer from their pains. It is then that the sad picture of suffering humanity ought to bring to his heart the first tenderness it ever experienced.
>
> (*Emile*: 222)

Reason is thus reunited with fervency, not through religious experience, but through an expression of love which Rousseau believed could be built upon the foundations of uncorrupted human nature by an unsullied imagination.

Rousseau and the problem of gender

Emile, this child of Rousseau's imagination, is male. Unlike Locke, who seemed relatively unconcerned with questions of gender, Rousseau regards each sex as having a specific and complementary role to play in the achievement of virtue. Indeed, without his mate, Emile is incomplete, a notion which the bachelor Locke, with his emphasis still more upon the heavenly rather than the earthly life, might have found rather odd.

From Rousseau's general condemnation of the corruptness of society, mothers are partly exempted. Theirs is a more natural relationship, especially to the feeding infant, and their closeness to their children makes them vital agents in child-rearing, even though the law (concerned with property not persons, and with peace not virtue) fails to give them their proper authority. Furthermore, contrary to common judgement, their instinct is generally correct.

> Mothers, it is said, spoil their children. In that they are doubtless wrong – but less wrong than you perhaps who deprave them. The mother wants her child to be happy, happy now. In that she is right. When she is mistaken about the means, she must be enlightened. Fathers' ambition, avarice, tyranny and false foresight, their negligence, their harsh insensitivity are a hundred times more disastrous for children than is the blind tenderness of mothers.
> (*Emile*: 38n)

Rousseau reintroduces gender as a significant factor in parenting. Genevieve Lloyd has demonstrated how, in the seventeenth century, reason became associated with maleness, it was seen as a skill whose achievement was associated with a more adult, more masculine way of understanding and dealing with the world (Lloyd, 1984: 38f). Increasingly in eighteenth-century thought, women are regarded as inhabiting a separate world of thought and feeling. This world is set in opposition to male rationality and sometimes is regarded as morally superior, but it is confined to the private domestic sphere and hence acquires a special relationship with childhood (ibid.: 57f).

It is not surprising, therefore, that Rousseau speaks specifically of mothering. His diatribe against wet nurses no doubt had something to do with the appalling rates of infant mortality associated with wet nursing, which were then coming to light in France, and also to emerging philosophical notions of an economy of the body (Garden, 1970; Donzelot, 1980), but Rousseau strives to make a more general moral issue out of the question. Using a nurse, Rousseau claims, leads the mother to encourage antithetical feelings in her child against the nurse who has fed him in an attempt to re-establish her place in the child's affections. But she cannot so easily reclaim the affections of her child.

> Instead of making a tender son out of a denatured nursling, she trains him in ingratitude, she teaches him one day to despise her who gave him life as well as her who nursed him with her milk.
> (*Emile*: 45)

This dereliction of duty by the mother is but the first step in undermining the family, a process of moral degeneration caused by a departure from nature. Relationships, thus, are defined in nature; the love between mother and child and the very vitality of the family depend upon the mutual love of mother and child and the reciprocal duties this generates.

When Sophie, Emile's intended mate, appears upon the scene in the fifth and final book of the *Emile*, it is to be educated for the specific role of wife and mother, a role essentially practical and unconcerned with abstractions, designed in all she does to please her man:

> What Sophie knows best and has been most carefully made to learn are the labours of her own sex. . . . There is no needlework which she does not know how to do. . . . She understands the kitchen and the pantry. She knows the price of foodstuffs and their qualities.
>
> (ibid.: 394)

But there is more to it than this: there is sex. In Sophie nature has become an art:

> Sophie loves adornment and is expert at it. . . . She has considerable taste in dressing herself up to advantage, but she hates rich apparel. . . . She is ignorant of what colours are fashionable, but she knows marvellously which look well on her. There is no young girl who appears to be dressed with less study and whose outfit is more studied. . . . Her adornment is very modest in appearance and very coquettish in fact. She does not display her charms; she covers them, but, in covering them, she knows how to make them imagined . . . and one would say that all this very simple attire was put on only to be taken off piece by piece by the imagination.
>
> (ibid.: 394)

Sophie is out to get her man for that is her whole purpose in life, but beyond marriage lies virtue and,

> Sophie loves virtue. This love has become her dominant passion. She loves it because there is nothing so fine as virtue. She loves it because virtue constitutes woman's glory and because to her a virtuous woman appears almost equal to the angels.
>
> (ibid.: 397)

The conservative nature of Rousseau's portrayal of the education of Sophie, contrasting as it does with the radicalism of his education of Emile, has occasioned a certain puzzlement amongst critics. One of the earliest, Mary Wollstonecraft, found herself exasperated by the notion of complementarity between father and mother, since in the everyday business of child-rearing, there can be no guarantee that the appropriate parent be will on hand at the right moment (Lloyd, 1984:

76). More recent feminist commentators have, not unexpectedly, also been critical (Okin, 1980; Badinter, 1981). He has been attacked as misogynist, and 'explained away' as a propagandist for the revolutionary bourgeoisie who elevated the nuclear family, and especially the mother within it, in opposition to the perceived degeneracy of the crumbling aristocracy. And at the heart of Sophie is her sexuality, the beauty of the feminine which both enslaves men and yet makes her man's servant; she is the antidote to reason and yet her grasp upon virtue is stronger than any man's. With Rousseau, gender is thrust to the centre of the educational agenda.

Judith Still has demonstrated that it is possible to read even the final book of the *Emile* sympathetically and with imagination, and, by so doing, to disclose the tensions which are a critical aspect of Rousseau's perception of the problems of human societies. This tension surrounds the problem of how, in an inegalitarian society, unequals may deal with each other justly. According to Still, Rousseau's answer is to take the concept of beneficence, a central issue for Enlightenment moral philosophy, and to rework it in terms of his own views on human motivation and the achievement of virtue. His discussion remains relevant, Still argues, because even in more egalitarian times beneficence is a central aspect of many relationships in late twentieth-century society, not least between, for example, parents and children, or teachers and pupils (Still, 1993: 2).

The problem in the writings of Rousseau, she suggests, is that whilst Rousseau reshapes the codes of beneficence in line with his own more egalitarian view of society, he maintains a rigid, hierarchical view of the relations between the sexes. For Rousseau, beneficence should work to overcome inequalities, not entrench them. The relationship it engenders should be dynamic, the benefactor motivated not by magnanimity, but by pity – that extension of *amour de soi* that allows love to grow. The beneficiary too should be able to respond, to imitate and become in turn a benefactor (ibid.: 30). Such a view of beneficence represents the perfect model of the parent–child relationship in which the child, as beneficiary, may grow in the love of the benefactor and in turn become active in the relationship; the interdependence being shaped by the dynamics of a changing relationship. The pleasure that Rousseau offers to the mothers who follow his advice is 'of seeing themselves one day imitated by their own daughters and cited as examples to others' daughters. 'No mother, no child,' he writes, 'between them the duties are reciprocal' (*Emile*: 46).

This utopian vision of reciprocal but dynamic interdependence is, according to Still, disrupted by what she terms a code of *pudicity* which Rousseau insists should regulate relations between men and women. By 'pudicity' (shamefacedness), Still means modesty as relating to the proper and chaste behaviour of women, and though there are good reasons why she avoids the more accessible word, it is perhaps easier to employ it here. Modesty, then, is the code (both of outward display and inner thought) which must regulate the behaviour of women. It holds women in a subordinate position to men and allows no room for the dynamic reciprocity which characterises his more general view of unequal interpersonal relations.

We have seen that, for Rousseau, reason is not sufficient motivation for human behaviour; passion is the driving force for human action, thought and feeling. Pity and sexual love are both passions which derive from *amour de soi* and are closely allied. Passion, diverted towards pity, leads to beneficence, but as sexual attraction it may become a destructive force; sexuality (regulated by female receptivity amongst animals) must be reserved and regulated in human society. The code of female modesty is that which controls sexuality, but reserve which is the essence of modesty can only confirm 'the integrity and stability of the unbreached and static self, whereas pity is dynamic and expansive, a movement out of the self towards the other' (Still, 1993: 82, 101).

Thus, the two codes of beneficence and modesty are on a collision course, though both are essential to the achievement of virtue in society:

> The benefactor . . . seeks to increase similarity and proximity between himself and the beneficiary: he offers gifts . . . he is hospitable (bringing about physical proximity), he shares his wisdom and experience. Pudicity, on the other hand, requires distance, separation, a strict enforcing of barriers and the maintaining of (sexual) difference.
>
> (ibid.: 106)

One way around this problem for the contemporary reader is simply to dismiss Rousseau's discussion of modesty as a patriarchal anachronism, and to see in his more positive, creative view of beneficence something that needs no check, no counter-force to control and reserve its power. Judith Still is primarily concerned with Rousseau's discussion of relationships between men and women, but she sees in the broad spectrum of Rousseau's writing a value to the code of modesty which would not be apparent from a superficial reading of those parts of the *Emile* which deal with Sophie.

The crux of this value lies in the darker side of beneficence which Still believes Rousseau was aware of, even if he did not articulate it clearly. There is the possibility that beneficence might be too intrusive in projecting *amour de soi*, through pity, upon another individual; it might gaze upon that which should be hidden and penetrate that which should be reserved (ibid.: 192). Amongst commentators, this unease has surfaced before in misgivings about the role of the all-powerful, all-seeing tutor in the *Emile*. Crocker, for example, accuses Rousseau of producing an automaton and Bantock objects to the production of a child unable ever to achieve maturity because it is never allowed to fail. Such readings fail, no doubt, to see the Enlightenment God figuratively represented in such figures as the Tutor – a rational and superior successor to the more arbitrary figure of Providence that haunted earlier writers – but, nevertheless, even if the power of the beneficent Tutor is reduced to human terms, it remains awesome and threatening (Crocker, 1973: 155; Bantock, 1980: 276; Charvet, 1974: 57; Still, 1993: 220).

Hence, the justice which Rousseau seeks through beneficence is precarious and the feminine, with its associated code of modesty, represents an attempt to preserve that precarious balance. It serves, as Still notes, to introduce an element of humanity, of struggle into the human society Rousseau attempts to create. Though Still is concerned with gender relations, it is not difficult to see the relevance of what she says to other unequal relationships in society, and to the parent–child relationship in particular. For whilst the beneficent relationship Rousseau envisages may, upon first inspection, appear an ideal model for the parent–child relationship, its oppressive potential should not be overlooked. The parental gaze, born of pity for the child's dependence, can be too penetrating, the generosity of beneficence too demanding. Nor, as the contemporary anguish over child sexual abuse demonstrates, can sexuality either be entirely ruled out of the parent–child relationship. The passion that inspires pity is never far from the erotic and the imagination that Rousseau insists is the faculty by which passion becomes pity, feeds upon the spectacle of innocence. Modesty, however, is not a defence which children naturally possess; like Sophie they must learn it as an art.

Parents deny the physical, sensual and even erotic nature of their relationship to childhood only with difficulty. Emotional possessiveness is its most obvious manifestation, and we have seen already various attempts to cope with its implications. Puritanism appeared to celebrate it through motherhood, only to deny it to fathers, and looked, instead, for a sublimation through religious ecstasy. Locke attempted to desiccate it with the rigorous discipline of reason, itself a code of modesty to prevent love overriding rationality. Rousseau glimpsed the tension and expressed it clumsily, even naively, in his description of the education of Sophie.

For all its bravado, the gaze that Rousseau turned upon the Sophie of his imagination was uncertain and occasionally voyeuristic in a way that was not evident when he created Emile. Rather like Locke, there are things which disturbed his settled image of the child. With Locke it was specific things like children's cruelty and perhaps, more generally, a resonance of Puritanism, and of the force of original sin which he could never shake off. With Rousseau, it was the perception of the power as well as of the necessity of passion, and of the thin line that divides pity from exploitation, virtuous love from encroaching desire. But when these disturbances are put to the back of the mind both Locke and Rousseau could banish the ghost of Pierre Bayle and paint a picture of childhood which captured its needs and its pleasures, and sensed the importance of the state of childhood for all humankind. It was in this that Rousseau especially made his contribution to Romanticism and its emerging conceptions of childhood:

> Love childhood; promote its games, its pleasures, its amiable instinct. Who among you has not sometimes regretted that age when a laugh is always on the lips and the soul is always at peace? Why do you want to deprive these little innocents of the enjoyment of a time so short which escapes them, and of a good so precious which they do not know how to abuse? Why do you want to fill with bitterness and pains these first years which go by so rapidly and can return no more for them than they can for you?
>
> (*Emile*: 79)

Chapter 4

The child of Romanticism I

The noble savage and romantic naturalism

> The whole ways and look of the child, so full of quiet wisdom, yet so ready to accept the judgement of others in his own dispraise, took hold of my heart, and I felt myself wonderfully drawn towards him. It seemed to me, somehow, as if little Diamond possessed the secret of life, and was himself what he was so ready to think of the lowest living thing – an angel of God with something special to say or do. A gush of reverence came over me, and with a single *good night*, I turned and left him in his nest.
>
> George MacDonald, *At the Back of the North Wind*

In discussing Puritanism and its approach to child-rearing, it was suggested that much of our contemporary understanding of the term came from its derogatory portrayal by writers associated with Romanticism and its nineteenth-century legacy. Here we shall explore the emergence of Romanticism as one of several influences affecting child-rearing and education in the late eighteenth and early nineteenth centuries. At about the same time, the evangelical revival gave new life to the dissenting tradition that had grown out of Puritanism, and a continuing belief in rational child-rearing, following Locke and later Rousseau, was also influential and not infrequently at odds with the ideals of Romanticism. We are faced, therefore, not with a clear cut progression of ideas, let alone any sense of the advancement of human wisdom, but rather with competing discourses that claim different histories and define themselves as much by opposition to other sets of ideas and beliefs as to their own intrinsic logic. To these complications must be added that which our own use of the word Romanticism brings. In relation to childhood especially, the bland view that Romanticism bequeathed to us the innocent child and swept away the doctrine of original sin has some limited measure of truth to it, but it scarcely begins to describe the tortuous journey the doctrine of innocence travelled, the blind alleys it went up, and the often disturbing lines of thought and expression it traversed. Even so, the doctrine of original innocence, and the immense value we place upon it, is undoubtedly central to late twentieth-century perceptions of childhood, and there is perhaps still nothing more significant to the way in which both public and private approaches to child-rearing are shaped. Even when the western world takes it upon itself to dictate to other societies how they should treat their children, the doctrine of childhood innocence looms large. It has possibly acquired a global significance far greater than the ancient Christian doctrine of original sin.

But there are even deeper resonances that flow, at least in part, from the legacy of Romanticism. Romanticism sought to heal the relationship between child and adult – that is to say the relationship between the child we were and the adult we have become – which the Romantics believed had been broken by the modernising drive of industrial capitalism. In so doing they gave an emotional definition to the concept of the self, which has scarcely been challenged (and, indeed, was reinforced by Freud), until post-structuralism began, late in the twentieth century, to probe questions of identity and subjectivity. Consequently this discussion entails a move away from a definition of the adult–child relationship couched in terms of child-rearing alone; rather parenting is turned upon its head. When we question our relationship to our own former selves, we find (or rather we have been taught to find) in our own childhood that which was the parent to our present state. It was the Romantics who taught us the importance of this trick.

In 1802 Wordsworth wrote the now famous line, 'The Child is father of the Man'. In 1993, Anthony Easthope, post-structurally and irreverently, put his own gloss upon Wordsworth's epigram by talking of his 'impossible desire that the subject make itself while writing Daddy out of the script' (Easthope, 1993: 44). Impossible the desire may well be, but the search for the integrated self will not be lightly given up. Rather than writing Daddy out of the script, the postmodern child seems set upon a programme which involves the total absorbtion into the self of Daddy, and Mummy and anybody else who gets in the way. To find a unity and harmony within the self is still regarded as the pinnacle of human happiness and it was that which Wordsworth sought, and subsequently so have most who have been touched by Romanticism's project.

More tangibly, Wordsworth's little epigram disturbs the parent–child relationship by finally accepting the inevitable – namely, that the only socialisation which counts is that appropriated by the child itself. Both Locke and Rousseau knew this, of course, but they clung to the hope that education would remain within the province of the adult, keeping the child in a state of suspended animation until years of reason and mature feeling should come. In Wordsworth is the final acknowledgement that no such suspension is possible. Some hundred years earlier, Pierre Bayle had mused upon the problems God initiated by deciding to reproduce the human race through the creation of babies and expressed his own scepticism about education; now the Romantics attempted a rescue less through education, which destroys the past, and more through memory which attempts to preserve it.

THE FEAR OF MASS SOCIETY

But there were also much less philosophical issues at stake. What gave rise to Wordsworth's anxiety over the relationship of child to adult was, in part, a more general anxiety about broader changes in the economic, social and political environment. In the course of the late eighteenth and early nineteenth century, demographic and economic change interacted with gathering momentum; in Levine's graphic phrase, 'Events were in the saddle and rode . . . mercilessly' (Levine, 1987: 141). The result was a younger and younger population reaching a peak in 1821 when almost four in ten of the population were under 15 years old, a feature that growing industrialisation and urbanisation must have made ever more visible (Wrigley and Schofield, 1981). Accelerating capitalism, however, was not without its benefits, giving rise to a new consumerism relating to childhood. For the upper and middle classes it was in toys, books and private education, whilst increased opportunities for wage earning amongst the women and children of the new urban proletariat may even have lead to increased spending on children, especially on their clothes (Plumb, 1975; McKendrick, 1974). But this took place against a growing perception of mass society which, for example, made London such an alienating experience for Wordsworth:

How oft, amid those overflowing streets,
Have I gone forward with the crowd, and said
Unto myself, 'The face of every one
That passes by me is a mystery!'

('Prelude' 1936: VII, 626–9)

Earlier, in the *Preface to the Lyrical Ballads*, in a passage remarkably prophetic of twentieth-century critiques of mass society, Wordsworth had bemoaned the blunting of powers of discrimination amongst readers of popular poetry, attributing this decline to 'the increasing accumulation of men in cities, where the uniformity of their occupations produces a craving for extraordinary incident, which the rapid communication of intelligence hourly gratifies' (Wordsworth, 1936: 735).

Mass society made its impact in other ways too. The French Revolution showed the mayhem that could be unleashed if political control failed and its shock waves may even have produced a certain fretfulness about childhood. In 1799 Hannah More complained that children had 'adopted something of that spirit of independence, and disdain of control, which characterise the times'. The 'times' were those, this indomitable lady feared, in which calls for the rights of man would lead to similar calls for rights for women and that 'the next stage of that irradiation which our enlighteners are pouring in upon us will produce grave descants on *the rights of children*' (quoted in Grylls, 1978: 196). Child-rearing had public, political as well as private domestic implications. There is a faint hint here, too, of a perception of children as a class, of a category who might disturb the social order. Of course, the children of the poor had been seen as a threat to the natural social order for a hundred years or more. The eighteenth-century Charity School and Sunday School movements and the Houses and Schools of Industry were designed to ensure that a judicious mix of labour and education kept the children of the poor from idleness (O'Day, 1982; Cunningham, 1991). Hannah More's principal concern was to bring to the children of the poor the socialising aspects of education which were available to the middle classes, but her efforts reflected also, perhaps, a more general concern about the young. The *individual* child had always been a threat to his or her own parents' peace of mind, but the notion that children as a class posed a threat, if only in Hannah More's imagination, does suggest a certain fretfulness about education and child-rearing, a loss of confidence in the Lockean principles which had achieved a certain orthodoxy in the eighteenth century.

Just as the Puritans had fretted about how to bring up their children in an irreligious world, the educated classes at the end of the eighteenth century began to fret about the preparation necessary for a child about to enter the disordered, rapidly changing world of their own time. They had more than Rousseau to prompt them to such thoughts. The theoretical opposition he had formulated between uncorrupted nature and polluted civilisation had become, it seemed, a reality. It was to be an anxiety, too, that grew through the early decades of the nineteenth century, as the middle classes slowly withdrew themselves and their children from the economic frontline and retreated behind the hedge, the shrubbery and the lawn into their suburban bunkers (Davidoff and Hall, 1987). Much has been made of the withdrawal of women from the public sphere, but their children went with them and this may well have increased the sense of the polarisation of the worlds of childhood and of (male) adulthood. As Spilka puts it, 'On the one hand . . . there is the long, insulated journey towards adulthood, and on the other, increasing complexities and difficulties, confusions and alarms, oppressive levellings and assorted blights, in the adult world itself' (Spilka, 1984: 162).

It was a relatively short step from this to a perception of childhood, not merely as a preparation for adult life, but as something with qualities of its own. The idea of a linear development, so characteristic of Locke, began to look less attractive. By the 1840s, with Rousseau's more sentimental ideas spreading, the belief that childhood had its own special capacities become a more commonplace observation. Andrew cites an anonymous commentator on children's fiction from the 1840s who claimed that,

> children are distinguished from ourselves less by an *inferiority* than by a *difference* in capacity – that the barriers between manhood and childhood are marked less by the progress of every power than by the exchange of many.
>
> (quoted in Andrews, 1994: 24)

Such remarks tell us much about the changes in perception which affected childhood in the late eighteenth and nineteenth centuries. No doubt most members of the emerging bourgeoisie just got on with the job of child-rearing as best they could, though some with a possibly kinder regard for their children's eccentricities. But seeping into their consciousness, perhaps allaying perhaps increasing their fretfulness, came a notion which was not new (indeed it was in some senses as old as Christianity itself), which imbued the child with mysticism and with power. In looking for coherence, for progress and above all for reason in human affairs, the Enlightenment had seen great promise in the malleability of the child, but little of virtue inhering in the state of childhood itself. But Romanticism, in rebellion against the coming of mass society, saw in childhood glimpses of a lost paradise. Wordsworth in particular turned to the fresh, unpolluted perception of the child of nature to repair a blunted sensibility, and the nineteenth century took up the notion in its own way, variously twisted it and turned it about to suit its own ends, but in general found the idea quite endearing.

THE CHILD OF ROMANTICISM

To understand Romanticism and its enduring significance for contemporary conceptions of childhood is to appreciate more fully what led to this perception of a polarisation of child and adult. And to see its growing influence upon the Victorian discourse of childhood, both in the public and in the private domestic sphere, is to begin to appreciate its enormous impact upon the cultural context within which childhood is viewed still in the twentieth century. If Puritanism left an enduring focus of opposition for liberal sentiments, and the Enlightenment a proposal for human progress which even now few can reject with conviction, Romanticism bequeathed many of those myths of childhood by which we imagine we understand the nature of the child and its behaviour. These are myths in Barthes' sense of the word; ideas of immense cultural power, whose significance is built up of layers of meaning, the origins of which have long been forgotten. Such myths appear now to be 'natural', to explain the world and its meaning for us, but their history, the conflict and confusions which surrounded their origins are now buried beneath an almost obsessive belief in their naturalness (Barthes, 1973). There is a politics to these myths of childhood which recent cultural and literary historians have begun to unearth. This politics is to be found in the opposition Romanticism voiced about ideas and practices concerned with both the place of reason and of religion in child-rearing. In voicing this opposition, the Romantics turned to nature as a source of inspiration dependent upon neither the human intellect nor religion as expressed through human agency.

Inevitably, as Spilka suggests, we tend to develop 'placard' notions of the opposition between Romanticism and the Enlightenment, with 'Nature-Feeling-Innocence-Childhood' on the one side and 'Society-Reason-Corruption-Adulthood' on the other (Spilka, 1984: 163). Rousseau is now, and indeed in the late eighteenth and early nineteenth centuries already had become, a victim of these over rigid distinctions. Yet it is his conception of nature and of the child's relationship to it which lies at the heart of Romanticism's own perception of the child. By the middle of the nineteenth century, claims Spilka, it was in England that Rousseau's conception of childhood was most strongly felt and 'most thoroughly domesticated', and the romantic figure of the man himself, dressed exotically in Armenian costume, best remembered (Spilka, 1984: 163). Eighteenth-century notions of sensibility had aligned nature not only with notions of feeling and imagination but also with reason. Hence for Rousseau there was no contradiction between an education based upon nature and one based on the pursuit of reason. Reason was not a sufficient basis for virtue, but in itself it was not wrong. However, Romanticism's fear of the growing utilitarianism of industrialised society – Blake's anger at the dark satanic mills that overshadowed his vision of Jerusalem – and growing anxiety about its consequences for the rapidly expanding urban areas of England, increased the yearning for a nostalgic rural past.

There is, as Spilka points out, a transition during the course of the early nineteenth century which translates the symbolic child from the rural to the urban context. The shift, however, is also from the abstract to the concrete. Both for the bourgeoisie struggling to establish themselves and their own rules of cultural reproduction, and for the urban proletariat (for whom the bourgeoisie were also busy devising rules of cultural reproduction), discourses about childhood acquired a public aspect. They became part of a political agenda of social reform. But this transition was accompanied by growing contradictions which stemmed, in part, from the way in which Rousseau's ideas became changed or lost their original impact. These ideas focused particularly around the child's relation to nature and to the way in which the conception of the child as noble savage changed as the reality of urban poverty and ignorance was brought to light (Cunningham, 1991; Andrews, 1994).

Some fifty years ago, in his study of Romantic naturalism and of the place of the noble savage within it, Fairchild argued that the late eighteenth- and early nineteenth-century wave of 'illusioned naturalism' involved not only the cult of scenery but also 'the cult of the child, the peasant and the savage'. Furthermore the child, the peasant and the noble savage began, in the Romantic imagination, to share characteristics in common; not least in their sense of wild freedom, in the way they drew virtue directly from nature and in so doing questioned the value of civilisation (Fairchild, 1961: 1). There is no space here to go into the origins and complex history of the concept of the noble savage, except to emphasise the way in which it was variously employed to probe and criticise the values and customs of civilised society. Its relationship to concepts of rationality was more ambiguous, though not as hostile as might be supposed. More specifically, the natural man of Rousseau's imagination was, in Lovejoy's phrase, 'a non-moral but good-natured brute' (quoted ibid.: 127). Emile, who represented for Rousseau the uncorrupted child of nature, was not in himself virtuous; rather he was free of the corruption that came with civilisation. In his infancy he was not to be swaddled and coddled and his diet was to be simple; as a child he learned to accept the hardships that nature confronted him with and this kept not only his body but also his mind keen and flexible. With a mind uninfected by civilisation, Emile could then observe civilisation and its absurdities and his innate sense of pity, uncorrupted by social manipulation, would be able to engage with the social world in pursuit of a virtuous life. Rousseau's child was not a primitive, invested with mystical virtues of its own, but rather a creature that possessed the innate potential to live a virtuous life if only an appropriate, uncorrupting education could be devised.

In terms of Rousseau's own impact upon ideologies of education and child-rearing, the process was slow and never uncontested. The earliest influence was, in fact, scarcely in tune with the sentiments of Romanticism, for in Rousseau's *Emile* some saw, or thought they saw, an education of nature that was as rational, as Christian and as morally utilitarian as anything Locke had to offer. Most infamously, Thomas Day became infatuated with Rousseau's Emile and, having failed to find a wife by more conventional means, attempted to raise a couple of female foundlings (renamed by him Sabrina and Lucretia) according to a curious mixture of supposedly Rousseauesque methods. Lucretia lasted only a year, and Sabrina too became unmanageable after he dropped hot sealing wax on her arm and fired pistols off next to her ear. She too had to be turned over to the care of others (Gaull, 1988; Coveney, 1967). Thomas Day did, however, write a story, *Sandford and Merton*, which was to enjoy popularity for much of the nineteenth century until, like so much early fiction and poetry for children, it was mercilessly parodied and destroyed by later Victorians.

Sandford and Merton is the tale of a spoilt child, Tommy, the son of the wealthy Mr Merton. He is sent to live with Harry, the sterling son of a yeoman farmer, Mr Sandford, who clearly understands the virtues of modest living and hard work. Both children come under the tutelage of Mr Barlow, whose surveillance of his charges matches that of Emile's own tutor. The story represents, in fact, a travesty of Rousseau's educational principles, since Mr Barlow fills his pupil's heads with knowledge not, as in Rousseau, entirely through direct experience of nature but second hand, through stories that Mr Barlow has the boys read aloud. Worse than this, since Tommy cannot read, Harry, apparently unaware of Rousseau's strictures on reading, teaches him, much to the approval of Mr Barlow.

But some perception of the noble savage did lie behind Day's story, albeit in 'a naturalised and domesticated form' (Andrews, 1994: 115). When Harry first visits the house of Tommy, Mrs Merton is disappointed by how little he is impressed by their obvious wealth. She suggests that Tommy give Harry a silver cup, but Harry rejects the gift on the grounds that he would worry about its being broken. Of the horn vessels he is used to, Harry happily confesses, 'ours at home are thrown about by all the family, and nobody minds it'. Childish prattle replaces the lofty scepticism about civilisation that Rousseau wished to develop in Emile. Thomas Day, however, was by no means the last writer for children to use the trick of the child whose honesty of expression exposes the follies of adult pretension.

With a much greater gift for storytelling but with not dissimilar principles was the Irish Maria Edgeworth, whose father had been an early disciple of Rousseau, and with whom she collaborated in her earlier ventures. In her story, 'The Orphans', published in the collection, *Parent's Assistant* of 1796, a young family, left destitute by the death of their mother and ejected from their home by an agent ('a hard man') of the English owner, take up residence in the ruins of a nearby castle. Living simply with nature, but employing great industry, native wit and above all extraordinary entrepreneurship, the children survive. Through their industry and honesty (and a little help from some gentry friends) they finally make it to prosperity and safety. But unlike Day, with his moral platitudes, Edgeworth's 'The Orphans' is rooted in a utility born of a real, if fictional, necessity. Even so, Edgeworth loses no chance to introduce sound factual knowledge. The children's making of rush candles, for example, prompts a long footnote quotation from Gilbert Whyte's *Natural History of Selbourne*, about whom Edgeworth comments to her child readers, 'no subject of rural economy, which could be of general utility, was beneath his notice'. It is, however, the entrepreneurial ingenuity of the young family that is breathtaking. Edmund, the only boy, full of inventive initiative, finds employment inside a gentry household. Unaccustomed to wearing socks and shoes, which creak and make his fellow servants laugh at him, he reports the problem to his older sister Mary in some distress. She promptly invents a new kind of house shoe made of cloth with a hemp sole. Not content with solving Edmund's problem, Mary is soon supplying the neighbourhood, and eventually Dublin itself. She is assisted by her two younger sisters and by Edmund himself and the division of labour devised is one Adam Smith, himself, would have been proud of.

'The child of nature', claims Bratton, 'is thus entrapped in the toils of utilitarian materialism' (Bratton, 1981: 43). But Bratton's is an unsympathetic judgement, itself clouded, perhaps, by Romantic sentiment. Maria Edgeworth is too good a storyteller for her fables not to make their point through the narrative; there is little need for pious platitudes. And her children are remarkably unoppressed by their situation: even if the power that nature gives them is turned to utilitarian purposes, it remains impressive. More important in Edgeworth is the spirit of Rousseau, a vision of children facing a corrupt and hostile world, but having gained a freedom of action which comes from learning driven by necessity, unfettered by the niceties of civilisation. Morality, too, is not entangled with manners, but is based upon simple reciprocity. Adult philanthropists stand apart, not interfering, and intervening only when required. This is the kind of tale that late twentieth-century children's rights lobbyists should have perpetually upon their desks.

But, claims Fairchild, Romantic naturalism wanted far more than that and in England, in particular, they made of Rousseau a more exotic figure. In any case the Romantic image of childhood did not depend upon Rousseau. The child of nature was already abroad. In the 1770s Anna Seward wrote a sonnet in which she depicted herself as a child who strayed 'With Infancy's light step and glances wild', a creature stirred by the wild landscapes of the deep Derbyshire dales,

> Romantic Nature to the enthusiast Child
> Grew dearer far than when serene she smiled.
> (Ashfield, 1995)

Almost thirty years later, in the hands of Wordsworth, the symbolism is far richer; the insouciant child with wild glances is no longer allowed such a casual relationship to nature. In his poem 'Three Years She Grew', Nature claims Lucy as Her own,

> Three years she grew in sun and shower
> Then Nature said, 'A lovelier flower

On earth was never sown;
This Child I to myself will take;
She shall be mine and I will make
A Lady of my own.

Myself will to my darling be
Both law and impulse: and with me
The Girl, in rock and plain,
In earth and heaven, in glade and bower,
Shall feel an overseeing power
To kindle or restrain.

Lucy dies and leaves to the poet only a memory of 'what has been/ And never more will be', but as Fairchild remarks Lucy represents the Wordsworthian and Romantic ideal of Nature, powerful and disciplinary perhaps, but a source of all human qualities; of beauty, of grace, of delight and of 'the breathing balm . . . the silence and the calm' that only Nature can give. Wordsworth was to claim for himself something of the same, although of a more masculine kind, in 'Tintern Abbey', finding,

In nature and the language of the sense
The anchor of my purest thoughts, the nurse,
The guide, the guardian of my heart, and soul
Of all my moral being.

(lines 108–11)

A few years after the turn of the century, Wordsworth was to produce his most definitive statement of Romantic childhood in the ode, 'Intimations of Immortality from Recollections of Early Childhood'. Here, claims Pattison, Wordsworth came closest to Rousseau, viewing childhood as 'both good in itself and, properly tended, the seed from which useful, fulfilled man is necessarily grown' (Pattison, 1978: 62). And as Coveney remarks, the ode became 'one of the central references for the whole of the nineteenth century in its attitude to the child' (Coveney, 1967: 81).

The sense of loss Wordsworth evokes in the opening stanzas of the poem is of a loss of the child's vision which had given to every 'common sight' of nature 'apparelled in celestial light,/The glory and the freshness of a dream'. The sight of a particular tree, a field remembered from childhood, even a flower at his feet, leaves Wordsworth mourning the loss of the fleeting vision that had once been his. At this point in its composition, the poem was to remain incomplete for some four years. When Wordsworth finally returned to it, he employed the myth of pre-existence to initiate a train of thought that strove to unite the child and its visions with the 'philosophic mind' of the mature adult. The 'trailing clouds of glory' which accompany the newborn child gradually fade away as the pleasures, labours, trials and ambitions of the earthly life fill the consciousness of the growing child. But, insists Wordsworth, something remains of this immortality,

High instincts before which our mortal Nature
Did tremble like a guilty thing surprised,

Those shadowy recollections,
Which, be they what they may
Are yet the fountain-light of all our day,
Are yet a master-light of all our seeing,
Uphold us, cherish and have power to make,
Our noisy years seem moments in the being
Of the eternal silence: truths that wake
To perish never.

(Stanza IX)

In the final stanza, Wordsworth appeals once more to Nature not to abandon him and once more there is the spirit of the Lucy poem, a sense of Nature's might and of her controlling power and of the intenseness of the relationship between Nature and humanity.

Thanks to the human heart by which we live,
Thanks to its tenderness, its joys, and fears,
To me the meanest flower that blows can give
Thoughts that do often lie too deep for tears.

(Stanza XI)

As Wordsworth himself acknowledged, relating the myth of pre-existence to childhood's special qualities was not new. In the middle of the seventeenth century the meditational poet Henry Vaughan had declared,

Happy those early days, when I
Shin'd in my Angel-infancy!
Before I understood this place
Appointed for my second race,
Or taught my soul to fancy ought,
But a white celestial thought.

('The Retreat')

But, as Pattison has argued, the tradition Vaughan represents is essentially a conservative one which sees individual human progress going from an almost false and delusory innocence in childhood to the decay and frustration of old age. It was this perception that caused Thomas Gray, not long before Wordsworth, to comment with some bitterness in his 'Ode on a Distant Prospect of Eton College':

> where ignorance is bliss,
> 'Tis folly to be wise.

Wordsworth, Pattison argues, is the culmination of a more radical tradition; one which rejected the oppressive tragedy of the fate of humankind, and saw, within some form of humanist education, the salvation of the human race. Such a tradition, he claims, can be found in Milton's Puritanism, in Locke's belief in reason and in Rousseau's belief in the education of nature (Pattison, 1978: 50). However, even within this more positive view of childhood, there can be no doubt that the child is seen to be in need of a restraining and a shaping force. Such, too, is the case with Wordsworth's Lucy, where Nature reserves the power to 'kindle or restrain'. In the ode, however, Wordsworth uncharacteristically strays beyond this belief in the shaping powers of nature, to imbue the child with a supernatural, immortal quality of its own. He himself wrote that,

> the visionary qualities of children have often been noted, and have been interpreted as intimations of immortality: I took hold of the notion of pre-existence as having sufficient foundation in humanity for authorizing me to make for my purpose the best use of it I could as a poet.
>
> (quoted Coveney, 1967: 77)

This somewhat defensive comment indicates that Wordsworth was not entirely at home with this manoeuvre, and Coveney, Pattison and Fairchild all point to this atypical aspect of his treatment of childhood.

Wordsworth's uncertainty points to the dilemma that always underlay the Romantic's elaboration of Rousseau and indeed, beyond that, explains the uncertain image of childhood that figures in the social reform movements of the early Victorian period (May, 1973; Cunningham, 1991). What may be justified, as Wordsworth claims, by reference to the poet's use of symbolic representations of humanity in the abstract, tends to look less attractive when confronting a real example of human infancy, especially if that infant is of the race of urchins, one of the urban poor. It is an old story that, as Wordsworth entered middle age, he became more conservative in his general outlook. Fairchild rather unkindly remarks that 'ecstatic praise of nature, enthusiasm for childhood and the mystic thrill of pantheism dwindle down to fumbling discourses on the factory system, national education and the Church of England' (Fairchild 1961: 187).

Certainly, Wordsworth's 'Westmoreland Girl' of 1845, a poem about a motherless lover of animals whose rescue of a lamb from drowning inspired the ageing poet, brought out of him a certain querulous anxiety about her relationship to the 'inferior creatures' and indeed to nature in general:

What then wants the Child to temper,
In her breast, unruly fire,
To control the forward impulse
And restrain the vague desire?

Easily a pious training
And a steadfast outward power
Would supplant the weeds and cherish
In their stead each opening flower.

Then the fearless Lamb-deliv'rer,
Woman-grown, meek-hearted, sage,
May become a blest example
For her sex, of every age.

Here is less the Romantic child than the daughter of the emerging bourgeois family described by Davidoff and Hall (1987) and Gorham (1982); a girl more suited to domestic suburban settings than to leaping into rivers to save young lambs, and one, furthermore, who must learn the difference between flowers and weeds! But it is unfair to see this simply as a narrowing of the intellectual imagination of an ageing poet. The relationship between the child and nature had always produced a discourse of some ambiguity. Neither Coleridge nor Blake, both more inclined to transcendentalism than Wordsworth, were content with the 'Immortality Ode'. Coleridge took exception to the weight of wisdom Wordsworth placed upon the child:

In what sense does [the child] read 'the eternal deep'? In what sense is he declared to be 'for ever haunted by the Superior Being', or so

> inspired as to deserve the splendid title of a mighty prophet, a blessed seer?
>
> (quoted Coveney, 1967: 87)

And Blake, on first acquaintance with the ode remarked, 'I fear Wordsworth loves nature, and nature is the work of the Devil. The Devil is in us as far as we are nature' (quoted Pattison, 1978: 65).

And as the Romantic child moved away from its rural origins and emigrated to the nineteenth-century urban shanty towns, the problem was by no means confined to Wordsworth. Andrews, for example, has demonstrated how far Dickens was exercised by the tension that inevitably lies between the attraction of Romantic symbolism and the unruly reality of the undisciplined child. Dickens' uncertainty about how to deal with real children was, Andrews argues, a response to the 'contradictions and confusions within the cult of primitivism', and to that heady combination of Rousseauesque belief in the natural innocence of children and Romantic conceptions of nature that had produced the 'Immortality Ode'. More than Wordsworth, however, Dickens had a clear enough sight of real children and the imaginative genius to know what belonged to fiction and what to the real world.

There were, of course, few more aware than Dickens of the symbolic power of the innocent child; of Nell and Paul Dombey (to mention but two of Dickens' catalogue of expiring children) dying so that a cruel and disinterested world might learn of its folly, of crippled Tiny Tim putting a brave face on his misfortunes and shaming the miser Scrooge, and of young David Copperfield, oppressed by the Puritan Murdstone, struggling so bravely for mental and spiritual survival. It is this, as Coveney remarks, that makes Dickens so significant an heir to the Romantic tradition and it was, above all, his great skill which enabled the child of Romanticism to be translated from the rural poetic scene to the grim urban one. He defended, too, the child's right to the development of its imagination against the utilitarian demand for an exclusive diet of fact in education. In an essay from *Household Worlds*, 'Frauds on the Fairies' written in 1853, he wrote,

> In a utilitarian age, of all other times, it is a matter of grave importance that Fairy tales should be respected . . . every one who has considered the subject knows full well that a nation without fancy, without some romance, never did, never can, never will hold a place under the sun.
>
> (quoted Gaull, 1988: 79)

In expressing such sentiments Dickens was fighting the same battle that earlier Wordsworth, Coleridge, Charles Lamb and later Kingsley fought against the moral and utilitarian rationalists; a defence of fairy tales and a plea for the value of the unfettered imagination against a belief in the necessity of realism, a dispute which haunts literature for children even in the late twentieth century.

Some have accused Dickens of inconsistency in his fictional treatment of children on the one hand and in his apparent approval of utilitarian methods of education for the poor on the other. Critics have seen in this the application of one law (Romantic) for the rich and another (moral and utilitarian) for the poor. There may be an element of truth in this but, argues Andrews, more significant is what caused Dickens to sense the tension between the demands of the child as perceived by the Romantic tradition and the demands of realism (Andrews, 1994: 3). Andrews claims that it was not Dickens' personal childhood experience that brought this tension into sharp relief, but his own perception of a very real tension at the heart of nineteenth-century England. In a rapidly industrialising and urbanising society, many social reformers were exercised by the need to exert control over the growing bands of street children, and yet at the same time their consciences told them that these very same urchins, who ran out of control through the streets of the big cities, were themselves industrialisations's prime victims. Cunningham (1991) and May (1973) have noted how mid-century reformers feared the precocity of the street children and strove to return them to their childhoods, but did so with the clear intention of re-ordering their lives under the most intense surveillance. The rural occasionally had attractions for health reasons and because of a sentimental view of family life that was still believed to exist there, but the freedom to sport with Romantic nature played little part in the social reformers' programmes.

THE FATE OF THE ROMANTIC CHILD

The development of the Romantic conception of childhood was complicated by far more than the existence of real children, however. In so far as the bourgeois family chose to incorporate it, it became not so much urbanised as domesticated. Late eighteenth- and nineteenth-century women's poetry is only just becoming more readily available in modern editions but merits particular attention because of the light it can throw upon the domestic scene (Ashfield, 1995; Breen, 1992;

Lonsdale, 1989). Seward's previously quoted vision of the wild Romantic child of nature provided a brief glimpse of the way women poets, too, connected the child with landscape and with nature, but of more specific significance are poems with a more domestic orientation. One example must suffice here.

Mary Robinson, for example, in an ode written on her daughter's birthday, 18 October, 1794, challenged that conservative tradition identified by Pattison in which the degeneration from infancy to old age is regarded as inevitable. The 'sad and toilsome road' of human existence cannot be eased by titles or power, she claims, rather:

> The balmy hour of rest alone, we find,
> Springs from that sacred source, Integrity of Mind!

'True Philosophy' can learn only from nature, not from 'Pedant's lore', in each season of human existence. Hence, even in 'Youth's ecstatic prime', her daughter can

> snatch from passing time,
> A wreath that ne'er decays!

Childhood, itself, should be a happy time:

> Then let it be the Child of Wisdom's plan,
> To make his little hour as cheerful as he can.

In the rejection of academic learning in favour of nature's teaching, in the search for individual integrity and in its positive belief in the value of children's happiness, the poem presents a Rousseauesque picture of childhood, but Mary Robinson goes further, conveying an almost Wordsworthian sense of continuity between child and adult. In her case, however, it is not the abstract child-as-father-of-the-man, but the sense of a tangible bond between mother and daughter in which the younger gives strength and peace to the older:

> Thou art more dear to me
> Than sight, or sense, or vital air!
> For every day I see
> Presents thee with a mind more fair!
> Rich Pearl in life's rude Sea!
> Oh! may thy mental graces still impart
> The balm that soothes to rest a Mother's trembling heart!
>
> (Ashfield, 1995)

Here is an all too brief glance at the potential power of the domesticated Romantic image, but its life was all too short according to Coveney:

> The purpose and strength of the romantic image of the child had been above all to establish a relationship between childhood and adult consciousness, to assert the continuity, the unity of human experience. . . . In later decades of the century, however . . . writers began to draw on the general sympathy for the child . . . to create a barrier of nostalgia and regret between childhood and the potential responses of adult life. The child indeed becomes a means of escape from the pressures of adult adjustment, a means of regression towards the irresponsibility of youth, childhood, infancy and ultimately nescience itself.
>
> (Coveney, 1967: 240)

This trenchant description of the growing decadence of the image of childhood in later Victorian literature must still be regarded as bearing some measure of truth. There is a sense in which Coveney is wrong to regard it as without precedent; Pattison identified a long tradition which viewed human progress from cradle to the grave as an inevitable journey to corruption, but Coveney is surely right to see the particular Victorian mutation both as a decadent form of Romanticism and also as something unhealthily sentimental and morbid.

A tension is evident in the work of George Eliot, for example, which shows just how problematic the Wordsworthian legacy proved to be. As a young writer in 1847 George Eliot had written a piece for a newspaper entitled 'The Wisdom of the Child'. In this she contemplated the nature of childish wisdom and found it in an imagined empathy between the child and Rousseau as they contemplated the wonders of nature:

> Thus, Jean-Jacques Rousseau, couched on the grass by the side of a plant, that he might examine its structure and appearance at his ease, would have seemed to a little child so like itself in taste and feeling, that it would have laid down by him, in full confidence of entire sympathy between them, in spite of his wizard-like Armenian attire.
>
> (Pinney, 1963:19)

But beyond this, George Eliot claims, the really wise distrust the moral corrosiveness of an unfettered enlightenment and in their self-imposed restraint accept what the dependent child has had to learn, the need to obey a higher law:

> Self-renunciation, submission to law, trust, benignity, ingenuousness, rectitude, – these are the qualities we delight most to witness in the child, and these are the qualities which most dignify the man.
> (ibid.)

The Wordsworthian origin of these sentiments is clearly pointed to by Eliot. The wise man,

> would be neither an angel, an anchorite, nor a saint, but a man in the most complete and lofty meaning of the name – a man to whom the 'child is father', perhaps in more senses than the poet thought; and who is no degenerate offspring, but a development of all the features of that heaven-born parent.
> (ibid.)

But whilst the sentiments of Eliot were Wordsworthian, the representation in her novels was not. Coveney has pointed out that her descriptions of children suffer from a lack of objectivity and lack the sense of irony so necessary to the successful portrayal of literary children; they lisp their way through childhood, tokens of a barely suppressed sentimentality. Thus Totty Poyser in *Adam Bede*:

> 'Mummy, my iron's twite told: p'ease put it down to warm.'
> The small chirruping voice that uttered this request came from a little sunny haired girl between three and four...
> 'Mummy, I would 'ike to do into de barn to Tommy.'
> (quoted Coveney, 1967: 165)

This points to a dilemma that affected much of the nineteenth-century discourse on childhood; that is to say a discrepancy between the sentiment and its representation. It is one thing to attribute to childhood human qualities as yet untarnished by society, it is quite another to be able to represent those qualities in literary children and to give them a strength and sense of realism. Dickens' children not infrequently suffered from the same problem.

Ashfield identifies a shift in the role of women poets from the dissenting and radical 'unsex'd' women of the late eighteenth century to the ideal of the female poetess emerging in the 1820s and 1830s, who agonised over the conflict between their creative instincts and the increasingly elaborate definition of their domestic role (Ashfield, 1995). Letitia Elizabeth Landon, for example, exhibited the influence of Rousseau in ways very different from Robinson. According to Ann Mellor, she strove to a achieve a femininity based upon Rousseau's description of the education of Sophie, part of an expression of femininity cultivated not only in the conduct books of the period, but also in a newer form of ideological propaganda to which Landon contributed extensively. These were annual gift books containing stories and verse, lavishly illustrated and sold to the young ladies of the bourgeoisie. The illustrations often presented women 'as chaste but none the less erotically desirable' or as 'the mother, devotedly attending the infant (usually titled) upon her lap' (Mellor, 1993: 112).

Landon's own vision of education, expressed in a poem called 'Children', is Rousseau filleted of every bone, Romantic without a hint of Nature's power and certainly a method that entails none of the restrictions put upon Sophie, or for that matter upon most of the daughters of the prudent middle classes:

A word will fill the little heart
With pleasure and with pride;
It is a harsh, a cruel thing,
That such can be denied.

And yet how many weary hours
Those joyous creatures know;
How much of sorrow and restraint
They to their elders owe!

How much they suffer from our faults!
How much from our mistakes!
How often, too, mistaken zeal
An infant's misery makes!

We overrule and overteach.
We curb and we confine
And put the heart to school too soon,
To learn our narrow line.

No; only taught by love to love
Seems childhood's natural task;
Affection, gentleness and hope,
Are all its brief years ask.

(Cole and Hope, n.d.)

In 1837 Landon wrote a fictive autobiography, *The History of a Child*, in which she presents herself as a solitary, sensitive child enduring 'the bitterness of neglect and the solitude of the crowd'. It is the history of a 'childhood which images forth our life' and repeats 'what it learned from the first, Sorrow, Beauty, Love, and Death' (quoted Mellor, 1993: 113).

The sentimentality of Landon and her successors is well preserved in a popular anthology, *The Thousand Best Poems* (Cole and Hope, n.d.). This includes hundreds of poems culled from the magazines and annuals of the Victorian era, many of them on domestic themes and presumably written by women, even though they were published anonymously. One such, entitled 'Papa's Letter', tells the tale of a little boy who has long golden hair after the manner of Hodgson Burnett's Little Lord Fauntleroy. His mother, busy writing letters and unwilling to be disturbed, pastes a stamp on his forehead and tells him to go and play at being a letter. Unfortunately, the child decides to post himself to his dead father in heaven:

'I'se a letter, Mr Postman,
Is there room for any more?

'Cause this letter's going to papa;
Papa lives with God, 'ou know;
Mama sent me for a letter;
Does 'ou fink that I tan do?'

Not receiving much encouragement from the clerk, he leaves the post office to be caught up in the busy crowd where the inevitable happens:

Suddenly the crowd was parted,
People fled to left and right,
As a pair of maddened horses
At that moment dashed in sight.

No one saw the baby figure,
No one saw the golden hair,
Till a voice of frightened sweetness
Rang out on the autumn air.

'Twas too late! a moment only
Stood the beauteous vision there;
Then the little face lay lifeless
Cover'd o'er with golden hair.

Rev'rently they raised my darling,
Brushed away the curls of gold,
Saw the stamp upon the forehead
Growing now so icy cold.

Not a mark the face disfigures,
Showing where a hoof had trod;
But the little life was ended –
'Papa's letter' was with God.
(Cole and Hope, n.d.)

Such verse speaks for itself in its capacity to draw upon a stock of emotional clichés to present stereotypical images of childhood's beauty which even the horse's hoof is not allowed to disfigure, and, not least, to grant its largely female audience a delicious pang of vicarious motherly anguish. But at least in 'Papa's Letter' there remains a plausibility in the context and concreteness in the detail. In another example, a poem called 'The Children We Keep' by a Mrs E.V. Wilson, the diaspora of sentiment into hackneyed metaphor is complete:

The children kept coming one by one,
Till the boys were five and the girls were three,

Like garden flowers the little ones grew,
Nurtured and trained with tenderest care:
Warm'd by love's sunshine, bathed in dew,
They blossomed into beauty rare.

Then two of the children die, not with the adventurous spirit that inspired 'Papa's Letter', but with a sickening disinclination to engage with anything, including life:

But one of the boys grew weary one day,
And leaning his head on his mother's breast,
He said, 'I am tired and cannot play:
Let me sit awhile on your knees and rest'.
She cradled him close to her fond embrace,
She hushed him to sleep with her sweetest song,
And rapturous love still lightened his face
When his spirit had joined the heavenly throng.

Then the eldest girl with her thoughtful eyes,
Who stood where the 'brook and the river meet',

Stole softly away into Paradise,
Ere the river had reached her slender feet.

The sentiment that perhaps best encapsulates Coveney's perception of the barrier that grew between childhood and adult life is expressed in the final lines of the poem where mother and father sit musing in later years after all the children have left home:

They talk to each other about the past,
As they sit together at eventide,
And say, 'All the children we keep at last
Are the boy and girl who in childhood died'.
(Cole and Hope, n.d.)

Such is the mould of decay that grew upon the Romantic image of childhood, but to accept Coveney's distaste for such sentiments is not to deny their significance or to belittle their power for nineteenth-century bourgeois society, and it is this emotion far more than that of Wordsworth or Mary Robinson that survives into the late twentieth century.

Chapter 5

The child of Romanticism II

The enemies of Romanticism

> O Lord, send thy Holy Spirit to cleanse our wicked hearts; and make us to love thee, O Lord God, and to love each other. Let us not despise poor people, but love them and help them; and let us not envy people who are greater or better than ourselves, but love them also, and bless them and do good to them. If any body is kind to us, give us hearts to be thankful to them and to love them: and if any body is unkind to us, give us hearts to forgive them, and love them too: for the Lord Jesus Christ prayed for the wicked people who nailed him to the cross. And, above all, make us to love our dear father and mother, and everybody who teaches us any good thing; and our dear brothers and sisters, and all the little children we play with: and may we never quarrel, as wicked men and devils do; but live in love like the angels of God in heaven.
>
> Prayer from Mrs Sherwood's *The Fairchild Family*, 1818

It is wrong to imagine that the child of Romantic naturalism was ever going to hold uncontested sway over the growing ranks of the English middle classes. There were other forces at work with a much stronger grip upon the means of influencing middle-class opinion. Rousseau was not only an inspirer of new ideas, but he also provided a target for those who wanted to create a moral panic about the state of society and about the education of children in particular. Was not Rousseau, after all, French? And look what had happened there in 1789. There is in the work of Thomas Day and even more in that of Maria Edgeworth an underlying democratic tendency, an implicit challenge to the established hierarchy, and in *The Orphans*, of course, the colonial English landowner's agent is the villain of the piece. This tendency was never seriously subversive in writing for children, but it was enough to cause Mrs Sarah Trimmer to register her distaste.

Mrs Trimmer was another turn of the century writer for children, committed to facts, but even more committed to religion. She was a self-appointed censor of fiction for children and like Hannah More she feared for the authority of parents. Her contempt for Rousseau was as absolute as her defence of Christianity. She was not evangelical after the manner of the Wesleyan tradition nor from the dissenting tradition of the Taylors, nor was she independent enough, like the Edgeworths, to enjoy radical possibilities. But from the centre of the Anglican establishment, she sought, in a periodical aptly named *The Guardian of Education* (1802–6), to root out subversion and in her own stories to radiate a rationality which left hierarchy undisturbed (Grylls, 1978; Salway, 1976). She had initially been lenient in her attitude to fairy tales (as long as children were given to understand that fairies were not real), but one correspondent to *The Guardian of Education* quickly took her to task on the question of *Cinderella*, which in the correspondent's opinion

> is perhaps one of the most exceptionable books that was ever written for children. . . . It paints some of the worst passions that can ever enter into the human breast, and of which little children should, if possible, be totally ignorant; such as envy, jealousy, a dislike to mothers-in-law and half-sisters, vanity, a love of dress etc. etc.
>
> (quoted Darton, 1982: 96)

As for nature, that is to be encountered only through walks attended by mother who carefully explains all that is to be properly learned, and though affection for animals is perfectly proper, it is so only within reason. For example, in the advertisement at the opening of later editions of her most famous stories, *Fabulous Histories Designed for the Instruction of Children Respecting their Treatment of Animals*, first published in 1786, she wrote,

> It certainly comes within the compass of *Christian benevolence* to shew compassion to the *Animal Creation*; and a good mind naturally inclines to do so. But as, through an erroneous education, or bad example, many children contract habits of *tormenting* inferior creatures, before they are conscious of giving them pain; or fall into the contradictory fault of *immoderate tenderness* to them; it is hoped that an attempt to point out the line of conduct, which ought to regulate the actions of *human* beings towards those over whom the SUPREME GOVERNOR has given them dominion, will not be thought a useless undertaking; and that the mode of conveying instruction on this subject which the author of the following sheets has adopted, will engage the attention of young

> minds and prove instrumental to the happiness of so many an innocent animal.

The 'following sheets' contain stories of a family of robins earnestly learning morality and manners whilst two children observing them learn from their parents to be kind to animals. It is interesting to note that, as with Locke, cruelty to animals is not put down to original sin but to ignorance or bad influence. However, the really significant feature of these stories is the way in which children are located in the hierarchy of the great chain of being. Indeed the whole book is infused with necessity of hierarchy, with the need for children to be at once benevolent to those beneath them (the animals), and deferential to those above them (parents). As the children's mother points out with sweet reasonableness,

> Children can do nothing towards their own support; therefore it is particularly requisite, that they should be dutiful and respectful to those, whose tenderness and care are constantly exerted for their benefit.

It is easy to mock Mrs Trimmer and, in the midst of radical ideas, rationalist or Romantic, stemming directly or indirectly from the influence of Rousseau, to dismiss her as an unthinking reactionary. But she repeats a growing orthodoxy about parenting and child-rearing, evident in Puritanism, codified by Locke and by no means absent from Rousseau himself: that the unequal relationship between adult and child must be regulated by both authority and tenderness on the part of the parent. The child must offer duty, loyalty and obedience, but like the animal has some claim upon the benefactor too. In the relationship of the children to the robins in Mrs Trimmer's hierarchical world is also to be found the essence of her ideal relationship between adult and child, a relationship which imposes a considerable responsibility upon the parents.

Mrs Trimmer was naive, clumsy and, like Hannah More, paranoid about corrosive influences coming over the water from France. Dickens was to get in his own jibe against their kind in *The Old Curiosity Shop*. Mrs Jarley, owner of the waxworks, hoping to attract members of the local boarding school for young ladies to her show, re-dresses her dummies and changes 'a murderess of great renown into Mrs Hannah More'. Miss Monflathers, the head of the said boarding school, is suitably impressed by the appearance in a waxworks show of such a worthy figure from the educational world (Chapter 29). But

Dickens' mockery comes some forty years after Sarah Trimmer and Hannah More first made their influence felt. At the turn of the century, they were both part of a much broader movement concerned with education and the reformation of manners (O'Day, 1982; Davido and Hall, 1987). Nor was Mrs Trimmer, for example, devoid of a sensibility towards the children of the poor, being herself caught up by the early revulsion against child labour in factories. 'I cannot', she says, 'think of little children, who work in Manufactories, without the utmost commiseration.' Faces, she wrote, which should bloom like roses are 'pale and sodden', limbs which should be robust are distorted, and tongues utter oaths 'which should be taught words of piety and virtue' (quoted Cunningham, 1991: 67). It is, in a sense, a tribute to writers like Dickens that twentieth-century commentaries upon the writings of people like Mrs Trimmer are, on the whole, so dismissive, and there is no doubt that in the last decade of the twentieth century, their preoccupations and methods strike us as odd. Nevertheless, there is a deep moral seriousness about their approach to children which carried the tradition of Locke, and before him of the Puritans and the Humanists, far into the nineteenth century.

Bratton has demonstrated how important publishing for juveniles was in the broad evangelical movement, not least in conjunction with the Sunday School Movement. To give the poor access to the Bible, they needed to be able to read and thus there was an important incentive for adults to attempt to communicate with children in appropriate language and narrative forms. The Religious Tract Society, founded in 1799 and including Hannah More amongst its writers, deliberately sought to use the hawkers of chap book and ballads as their means of distribution, disguising moral tracts by using titles that would not distinguish them from the hawkers' more usual wears. The Society was also prepared to undercut the prices of rival publications. It also gave new life to that classical Puritan tract, Janeway's *A Token for Children*. The Society for the Promotion of Christian Knowledge, an organisation dating from the late seventeenth century and much involved in schooling during the eighteenth also, turned more of its attention to publishing in the nineteenth century, taking on some of Mrs Trimmer's work in 1814 as its first venture into juvenile fiction (Bratton, 1981).

As Davido and Hall have shown, this broad evangelical movement was influential in laying the foundations for middle-class domestic life in the nineteenth century (Davido and Hall, 1987). Anne and Jane Taylor's mother, for example, wrote several domestic treatises, the inspiration for which no doubt came partly from her own experience of running a household, but she also acknowledged debts to other writers including Hannah More and Maria Edgeworth. To her, mothering was like running a business and should be conducted rationally and with a proper sense of order. Within those constraints, however, time should always be found to listen to children who should be treated with respect and kindness, and taught to share the joy and love of religious faith. It is impossible to encounter the Taylor family and not to feel that their own family achievement was very considerable, but the dividing line between a religious belief that produces warmth and love and one that appears cold and oppressive is very fine, and the increasing use in the twentieth century of the term Puritan to describe almost any religious influence upon child-rearing clouds our perception even more.

THE PURITAN LEGACY

'Puritan' had always been used as a term of political abuse, but it is only in the later nineteenth century that the label seems to emerge specifically to denigrate methods of child-rearing. It is worth bearing in mind that Susanna Wesley, that most famous of 'Puritan' parents (though the child of a dissenting minister persecuted for his beliefs), herself joined the Church of England and married one of its ministers. Furthermore, the evangelical revival that her sons John and Charles were so closely associated with through their Methodism was as broad a religious movement as Puritanism had been in the late sixteenth century. In any case there is evidence that Susanna's child-rearing methods were not entirely successful. For example, the will of her daughter, Mehetabel (Hetty) was clearly never broken. She was as determined as her mother, and refused to play the dutiful daughter. In her twenties she repeatedly frustrated her parents' attempts to find her a husband, eventually became pregnant by some unknown lover and was hastily married off to a plumber and glazier, beneath her in status and education. Subsequently she lived an embittered if eventually contrite life, railing against loveless marriage (Lonsdale, 1989).

In 1733, she also left the world a poem written to her own dead baby, an 'Infant Expiring on the Second Day of its Birth', which begins,

> Tender softness, infant mild,
> Perfect, purest, brightest child;

Transient lustre, beauteous clay,
Smiling wonder of the day:
Ere the last convulsive start
Rends the unresisting heart;
Ere the long-enduring swoon
Weighs thy precious eyelids down
Oh! regard a mother's moan,
Anguish deeper than thy own!
(quoted in Lonsdale, 1989)

When Susanna was writing to John in 1732 about her child-rearing methods, she was describing the order and discipline required to prevent a household containing possibly more than a dozen children at any one time from descending into chaos. The following year, her daughter, writing a poem during her confinement, was contemplating the loss of the creature she had just given birth to. It is dangerous to generalise attitudes to childhood without taking note of circumstances.

Nevertheless, Lawrence Stone is able to find a line of continuity from seventeenth-century Puritanism, through Susanna and John Wesley to those like Hannah More and Mrs Trimmer at the end of the eighteenth century, a connection between 'the caring but authoritarian discipline of the Puritan bourgeois parent' and that of the 'Evangelical bourgeois parent'. It is also true that the evangelicals, like the Puritans, railed against the perceived laxities of their age and sought morality, not so much through spirituality as within the disciplined life of the family. John Wesley, in 1783, complained in his *Sermon on the Education of Children*, that only one in a hundred parents were now prepared to break the will of their children, to bring them to submit to their parents so that they might from that learn submission to God (Stone, 1979: 294).

There are examples, too, in the nineteenth century of what Coveney calls 'religious savagery' (1967: 34). Two examples must suce here; one from the world of children's books, the other a very real incident from America. By the early nineteenth century, writing for children was well established and Mrs Sherwood wrote within the didactic, moralising tradition established by writers such as Hannah More and Mrs Trimmer. Her stance on original sin, however, was particularly partisan:

> All children are by nature evil, and while they have none but the natural evil principle to guide them, pious and prudent parents

> must check their naughty passions in any way that they have in their power, and force them into decent and proper behaviour and into what are called good habits.
>
> (quoted Darton, 1982: 169)

Mrs Sherwood's story of *The Fairchild Family*, begun in 1812 whilst she was in India and much associated with missionary activities, contains a notorious example of what she expected prudent parents to do. Mr Fairchild finds that his children have been squabbling with each other about a doll and decides upon a lesson that will, he hopes, encourage them to 'pray more earnestly for new hearts, that they may love each other with perfect and heavenly love'. In order to achieve this worthy objective, he takes them on a walk through a dense wood to a ruined house. The children are suitably frightened but are reassured by their parents that no harm will come to them. Then, as they approach the house, they encounter their object-lesson,

> Just between that and the wood stood a gibbet, on which the body of a man hung in irons: it had not yet fallen to pieces, although it had hung there some years. The body had on a blue coat, a silk handkerchief round the neck, with shoes and stockings, and every other part of the dress still entire: but the face of the corpse was so shocking, that the children could not look at it.
>
> (from Chapter 'On Envy')

The hanged man had killed his brother and thus provided a suitable lesson for the Fairchild children of the appalling consequences of unchecked sibling rivalry. Not surprisingly, the children knelt and prayed for new hearts not prone to envy, much to the approval of their father. Another lesson satisfactorily learned, it would seem, though, as Darton mischievously points out, the Fairchild children never do seem to learn (Darton, 1982). It is also, perhaps, worth pointing out how patient Mrs Fairchild is, and how much she meets Mrs Taylor's demands that time should always be found for children. Mrs Fairchild has a patience and sympathy with her erring offspring quite at odds with the pompous moralising of their father.

In America, a few years later, Francis Wayland, a Baptist minister and college president, also expressed strong views about the rearing of children:

> The notion that a family is a society, and that a society must be governed, and that the right and duty of governing this society rests with the parent, seems to be rapidly vanishing from the minds of

> men. In place of it, it seems to be the prevalent opinion that children may grow up as they please, and that the exertion of parental restraint is an infringement upon the personal liberty of the child.
>
> (quoted by McLoughlin, 1975: 22)

Wayland was another product of the religious revival. His father, an emigrant from England, had become a Baptist minister following a profound religious experience. He was eventually followed in his vocation by both his son and grandson. Obedience of child to parent was pivotal to their moral doctrine and thus was also essential to Francis Wayland's own practice as a parent. In 1831 he wrote, anonymously, to *The American Baptist Magazine* to recount an incident involving himself and his then 15-month-old son. The infant had for some time been showing signs of growing independence. What provoked the incident in question was a show of temper before breakfast one Friday morning when Wayland took him from his nurse's arms. The child was holding a piece of bread at the time and Wayland took it from him until he calmed down. When he did stop crying his father offered him the bread again, but this only produced another show of temper. Wayland decided that now was the time to insist upon obedience. He put the child on his own in a separate room and every hour or so went to offer him the bread and to take him in his arms. The child refused and went to bed without food. It was 10 o'clock the following day when he finally took the bread and some milk from his father, but would still not allow his father to pick him up. Wayland continues,

> About one o'clock Saturday, I found that he began to view his condition in its true light. The tones of his voice in weeping were graver and less passionate, and had more the appearance of one bemoaning himself. Yet when I went to him, he still remained obstinate. You could clearly see in him the abortive efforts of the will. Frequently he would raise his hands an inch or two, and then suddenly put them down again.

At 3 o'clock the conflict was finally ended:

> To my joy, and I hope gratitude, he rose up and put forth his hands immediately. The agony was over. He was completely subdued. He repeatedly kissed me, and would do so whenever I commanded. He would kiss any one when I directed him, so full of love was he to all the family. Indeed, so entirely and instantaneously were his feelings

> towards me changed, that he preferred me now to any of the family. As he had never done before, he moaned after me when he saw that I was going away.
>
> (quoted McLoughlin, 1975)

Such extreme examples, literary or real, should be regarded with care. Darton comments of Mrs Sherwood's *The Fairchild Family* that, whilst popular and widely read during the nineteenth century, it was also 'as completely ridiculed, and as honestly condemned by child-lovers, as any English book ever written for children' (Darton, 1982: 170). Subsequent editions of the *Fairchild* history successively modified the original, until by the end of the century, the grotesque power of the earliest stories was, as Grylls puts it, 'dexterously gutted' (Grylls, 1978: 91). In any case, as L.B. Lang had already pointed out in 1893, it was a considerable error to stereotype Mrs Sherwood as the pious spinster of restricted upbringing and education, who had no real understanding of children. In fact Mrs Sherwood, by her own account, had quite an extensive and liberal education and, as a young adult, had opportunities to meet many of the cultural elite of her day. Once married she not only had children of her own, but, whilst in India, adopted others, set up schools and worked tirelessly for the welfare of all the children associated with her household. Her own upbringing was certainly strict and disciplined, but perhaps most interesting is the revelation that, like the Taylors, she and her siblings enjoyed a rich fantasy life of their own making in their nursery, writing stories, reading romances and acting out scenes from *Robinson Crusoe* (Lang in Salway, 1976). Bratton, too, offers a vigorous defence of Mrs Sherwood stressing the way in which she takes children as 'entirely serious as moral beings', commenting upon the story's reception in some quarters, that

> It was only those adult readers who were increasingly solicitous of childish sensibility, or in evangelical terms were so foolish as to put their children at risk by sentimentally concealing from themselves the inevitability of original sin and infant corruption, that complained of the book.
>
> (Bratton, 1981: 56)

Francis Wayland, too, sparked off a storm of protest. What seems to have caused particular offence was his 'philosophising' about what appeared to less intellectually minded people as a simple act of brutality. But at least his actions spawned a wicked piece of doggerel by way of riposte. It was published in *The Literary Subaltern*, and included the following two stanzas.

> And then I shut him up again to try his little spunk –
> Exhausted nature soon gave way and he began to funk,
> And then quite starved and wan and faint, he begged me for his
> supper,
> And as I'd carried all my points, I gave him bread and butter.
>
> For what I've done, and mean to do, to every wicked boy,
> And tell the tale to all the world and fill men's souls with joy;
> And now my darling boy has got the means of grace,
> I'll let him look upon the world and scorn the human race.
> (quoted in McLoughlin, 1975)

Two of the lines of criticism implicit in these sentiments are worth noting. The first stanza scorns the assumed rationality of Wayland's act – that it should be seen as an argument (with a 15-month-old child) in which points are won and lost. The second suggests a humanist critique of an arrogant religiosity which scorns the unredeemed mass of humankind. Without at all wishing to suggest that the anonymous poet was doing more than poking fun at a grossly over-serious and ill-proportioned response to a trivial incident, these two criticisms do have a certain significance to them. First, the 'poet' criticises the failure to appreciate the childish nature of what the little infant did, a failure to distinguish between an act of principle and a childish reflex – a simple lack of common sense in interpreting the meaning of the child's behaviour. Second, there is a sharper social criticism of religious child-rearing as something which is exclusive in its desire to separate the saints from the rest of humankind. There is actually something quite sophisticated in this knock-about humour, something which suggests that child-rearing really had entered the public domain as an issue which could provoke heated debate.

ROMANTICISM AND THE CRITIQUE OF PURITANISM

The history of religious influence upon child-rearing is insidiously rewritten in the nineteenth century by an increasingly antagonistic and sentimental Victorian Romanticism. That it is difficult now to take Isaac Watts seriously is not only because of the cultural distance that lies between him and us (though that, of course, is considerable), nor because of the wit of the irreverent Lewis Carroll (damaging though that is to reputations); it is also because the conception of childhood and the nature of the adult–child relationship that is implicit in the Puritan tradition has been anathematised by the intervening cultural force of Romanticism. It was a force of more power than coherence perhaps, and driven more frequently by anger than by reason. Nevertheless, its anti-Puritan invective has produced one of the most significant myths of the twentieth-century Anglo-Saxon world.

In the hands of Dickens, for example, religion becomes not a focus of domestic striving (as with the real Taylor family, for example), but rather an inevitable source of oppression (Adrian, 1984; Andrews, 1994). Take, for example, Arthur Clennam in *Little Dorrit*.

> There was the dreary Sunday of his childhood, when he sat with his hands before him, scared out of his senses by a horrible tract which commenced business with the poor child by asking him in its title, why he was going to Perdition?. . . . There was the sleepy Sunday of his boyhood, when, like a military deserter, he was marched to chapel by a piquet of teachers three times a day, morally handcuffed to another boy. . . . There was the interminable Sunday of his nonage; when his mother, stern of face and unrelenting of heart, would sit all day behind a Bible – bound like her own construction of it, in the hardest, barest and straightest boards, with one dinted ornament on the cover like the drag of a chain, and a wrathful sprinkling of red upon the edges of the leaves – as if it, of all books! were a fortification against sweetness of temper, natural affection, and gentle intercourse.
>
> (Chapter 3)

This was the routine oppressiveness which Dickens found so antithetical to his vision of childhood. In *David Copperfield* it is also striking that, in his portrayal of Murdstone, Dickens needs to explain so little about Murdstone's religious orientation to invoke the myth of a repressive Puritanism. Equally, the name of the school to which the young David is sent, Salem, was probably already sufficient in itself to connect nineteenth-century evangelicism with the tarnished image of late seventeenth-century New England Puritanism, and with Morgan's 'preposterous land of witches and witch hunters, kill-joys in tall-crowned hats' (Morgan, 1958: xi).

The major landmarks which further chart this mythologising of religious childhoods are well established literary monuments which need only brief comment. George Eliot's *Silas Marner* tells of a man, ruined by a treacherous religion, redeemed by the female child of Romanticism, complete with golden curls. Mention has been made earlier of the problems Eliot had in representing children, and the children in *Silas Marner* are no exception. This, however, only emphasises the power the Romantic myth of childhood had acquired by 1861 when the novel was published; that a symbol described in clichés could carry such emotional weight. Of particular significance is that the child rescues the man, not from drink and debauchery, but from the destructive consequences of a Puritan childhood. Silas comes from 'that little hidden world known to itself as the church assembling in Lantern Yard', a member of 'a narrow religious sect' which is the centre of his life. Silas, however, is accused of theft, and the church which framed and gave significance to his youth and early manhood fails to perceive the innocence behind his seeming guilt. Far from being able to read morals from behaviour, the church resorts to prayer and the drawing of lots to establish guilt, rejecting reason in favour of a dark world that meddles with unknown forces. Fleeing from this treachery to isolation, anonymity and obsessive miserliness, Silas reaches his nadir when his gold is stolen from him. Redemption comes through the adoption of an infant girl whose mother dies leaving her, apparently orphaned, at his cottage door. Her golden curls replace the stolen gold, and her innocence and devotion gradually draw him back to life and sociability. As he, under his adopted daughter Eppie's guidance, re-enters the world, so that of Lantern Yard is literally destroyed, buried under the building of a new factory. Silas is left to learn the wisdom of the child, and to accept that much that was dark about his old religious life will always remain so. Dolly Winthrop, a neighbour, provides the moral:

> It's the will o' Them above as a many things should be dark to us; but there's some things as I've never felt i' the dark about, and they're mostly what comes i' the day's work.

And Silas learns the lesson:

> Since the time the child was sent to me and I've come to love her as myself, I've had light enough to trusten by; and now she says she'll never leave me, I think I shall trusten till I die.

Thus the nineteenth century provided its own literary critique of narrow-mindedness and bigotry, of rigid and unfeeling forms of child-rearing, and associated them with a kind of generic Puritanism (Sommerville, 1992: 15). Semi-autobiographical and autobiographical work written later, like Samuel Butler's *The Way of All Flesh* of 1903, and Edmund Gosse's *Father and Son* of 1907, reinforced this critique of religiously motivated child-rearing. If *Silas Marner* embodied the Romantic critique of Puritanism, Butler and Gosse provided a commentary upon it. Indeed Gosse claimed his book to be 'the diagnosis of a dying Puritanism', and Butler provided a historical sketch of family relationships which explicitly laid the blame for the state of early nineteenth-century parent–child (or, more specifically, father–son) relationships at the door of the Puritan tradition:

> In the Elizabethan time the relations between parents and children seem on the whole to have been more kindly. The fathers and sons are for the most part friends in Shakespeare, nor does the evil appear to have reached its full abomination till the long course of Puritanism had familiarised men's minds with the Jewish ideals as those which we should endeavour to reproduce in our everyday life. What precedents did not Abraham, Jephthah, and Jonadab the son of Rechab offer? How easy was it to quote and follow them in an age when few reasonable men or women doubted that every syllable of the Old Testament was taken down *verbatim* from the mouth of God. Moreover, Puritanism restricted natural pleasures; it substituted the Jeremiad for the Paean, and it forgot that the poor abuses of all times want countenance.
>
> (Chapter 5)

Both Butler and Gosse clearly felt that Puritanism lay in the past, and Grylls is surely right to argue that neither book is anti-Victorian in its attack upon Puritan attitudes to child-rearing. Rather both books are 'quintessentially Victorian', presenting the Romantics' critique of Puritanism, not from the heat of the battle, as did Dickens, but from a position which suggests that the battle was already won (Grylls, 1978: 153).

Nearly a hundred years after the publication of Butler's and Gosse's condemnations of Puritan parenting, there is a tendency to appropriate their critique as if it were our own, and furthermore to assume that in so doing we are criticising the Victorians. But, in any case, how just was their condemnation? Their own accounts (veering between fiction and autobiography), and the examples of Francis Wayland and Mrs Sherwood, might encourage us to think they were right. But some 200 years ago, the Taylors lived a deeply religious life, highly disciplined and intensely demanding of both parents and children. It was not the kind of life imposed upon the fictional Arthur Clennam, but one which fostered development through play as well as prayer and hard work. Ann and Jane, in particular (to say nothing of the dreaded Mrs Sherwood herself), indulged in the kind of imaginative play associated with the much more famous Brontë children. At the same time, the Taylors learnt the duties of a housewife, the skills of the engraver and, above all, the value of religion as a defence against a potentially hostile world.

THE VICTORIAN CHILD

'Victorian responses to children', comments Grylls, 'were the product of two quite different intellectual traditions. One was broadly the legacy of Rousseau; the other of John Wesley. Coiled together, these two traditions could create weird patterns of thought' (1978: 23). The legacy of Rousseau itself was far from simple, embodying as it did both rationalist and Romantic tendencies, and the broad evangelical movement encompassed a wide range of approaches to child-rearing. It is perhaps not so odd, given the complexity of these intellectual strands, that the twentieth century has constructed Victorian parenting as uniformly strict, oppressive even, and patriarchal, whilst at the same time believing this same context to be the one in which the child of Romanticism flourished.

Whilst Romanticism's attack upon the rationalist tradition of the Enlightenment was, as we have seen, ambiguous and half-hearted, always prepared to come to some accommodation in the face of 'real' children, its campaign against Puritanism was never other than intense and never averse to a little emotional blackmail. The following verse, 'Let Them Laugh and Play', by 'E.T.' could be addressed to any mother inclined to heed Susanna Wesley's advice about keeping the children quiet:

> Parents, when you hear your children
> Laugh and shout in childish glee,
> Do not let the noise annoy you,
> Even though you harassed be.

And to any inclined to question this injunction, the stern answer comes,

> I have seen the eyes of parents
> Wild with tears they could not shed,

Bending in distracting sorrow
O'er a darling's suffering bed.

The poor mother can but offer contrition;

Once she told me, that their noises
Almost crazed her aching head,
While she shadowed every frolic
By the hushing words she said;
'Now,' she cried, 'could I but hear them
Bounding round in merry glee,
Could their voices break the stillness,
What a mercy it would be!'
(Cole and Hope. n.d.)

But if one looked for a Victorian orthodoxy about parenting, it would not be Romantic in its conception. In so far as generalisation is possible, the prevailing doctrine could probably best be described as a rational evangelicism with a softening in tone during the course of the century; certainly this is what the many advice books on child-rearing would suggest (Beekman, 1978; Hardyment, 1984; Kincaid, 1992). Kincaid, especially, shows how easily a rational evangelicism could absorb notions of childhood innocence, when innocence was defined as a lack, an emptiness that had to be filled with care (1992: 87–95). Nor was it difficult to incorporate and domesticate Nature itself. Wordsworth's Nature, epitomised by the awesome, black mountain peak that 'with a purpose of its own/And measured motion like a living thing' so frightened him as a boy, sinks easily into the lake of bourgeois tranquillity with scarcely a surface ripple ('Prelude', Book I: lines 383–4). The wild Derbyshire dales that excited Anna Seward as a child turn into the cultivated suburban garden in which the child grows and is nurtured by mother's watchful surveillance.

Indeed for the bourgeois child, Nature *becomes* the garden as this acquires a growing significance towards the end of the century. For adults it becomes the lost paradise of childhood happiness, for children a place to nurture and express innocence. The enduring strength of that image is nowhere clearer than in Frances Hodgson Burnett's *The Secret Garden*, published in 1911, a garden where the orphaned and embittered Mary Lennox and her supposedly crippled cousin, Colin, regain both mental and physical health with the help of Dickon, a child of nature, and his entourage of wild (but very tame) animals. Their return to childhood in the secret garden eventually allows the return of Colin's father from a self-imposed exile inflicted after the death of his child-like wife in the self-same garden.

The myth of the garden lingers far into the twentieth century but becomes associated with a sense of loss, of yearning for a past that can never be quite recaptured. One of its most poignant expressions is as late as 1958 in Philippa Pearce's *Tom's Midnight Garden*, in which Tom, sent away from his own family because of illness, finds himself cooped up in his uncle and aunt's tiny flat with nowhere to play. He discovers solace and friendship with a girl in a garden, a garden which he can only enter at the dead of night when the clock strikes thirteen. But the girl, Hetty, grows older in later visits to the garden and Tom, caught in his own childhood, can only watch as she fades away. There are distant echoes of early Romanticism here; the garden, as nature somehow surviving the destructive march of the urban, is still a place of beauty and of mystery with a power to oer comfort and to regenerate. But real life is on the outside, beyond and after the garden, and Tom's distress at losing Hetty is only resolved when he discovers that she is in fact the old lady who owns the house, now divided into flats. It was the strength of the old lady's memories of her own none too happy childhood which allowed Tom to find the old garden, long since built over. Hetty's memories, her own recollections of the comfort she found in the garden, uniting her in old age with her childhood, give Tom respite from the barrenness of the urban backyard and allow him a glimpse of nature. Not only nature in its domesticated form finds expression here, but also that other legacy of Romanticism – the significance of childhood for adult memories. It is also worth observing that, whilst adult fiction and poetry tended to flounder in their representation of the Romantic child and turned to a sentimentality with often dubious overtones, children's fiction found a way of locating the child in nature, and, through fantasy, of preserving that sense of the depth of childhood experience which inspired Wordsworth.

From the Puritan side, the doctrine of original sin ends not with a bang but a whimper, lapsing into irrelevance or rather, according to Briggs, merging with Romanticism and evolving into theories of recapitulation in which the primitive, the child, has to evolve into the civilised adult (Briggs, 1995: 169; Cunningham, 1991: 123–32). The more exotic versions of this doctrine were shunted o into quiet educational backwaters where they still exist today in the alternative educational programmes of the Rudolf Steiner schools. However, as Kincaid points out, some rough and ready theory of recapitulation made it possible to hold onto the idea of the moral inadequacy of childhood without abandoning the educational aim of improvement. Hence Thomas Arnold in his heroic eorts to shape religion as a force for civilisation through the English public school wrote,

> my object will be, if possible, to form Christian men, for Christian boys I can scarcely hope to make; I mean that, from the natural imperfect state of boyhood, they are not susceptible of Christian principles in their full development upon their practice, and I suspect that a low standard of morals in many respects must be tolerated amongst them, as it was on a larger scale in what I consider the boyhood of the human race.
>
> (quoted Kincaid, 1992: 71)

The evangelical tradition slowly lost the pre-eminent place that it held at the turn of the century and with it the significance of the doctrine of original sin lost its potency. Maybe the patriarchal Victorian father did to some degree replace the vengeful God of Puritanism, but he is a poor, confined, domesticated figure, marginalised in a way that Mrs Sherwood's Mr Fairchild would never have tolerated. Parental and especially patriarchal authority needed the support of a proximate God to make the claims Gosse and Butler found so irksome. Perhaps, as Grylls suggests, the real loss to children of this decline was a reluctance to treat them with the moral seriousness so characteristic of the early evangelical tradition (Grylls, 1978: 197). Treating children as innocent may grant them more freedom to develop in their own way and at their own time, but it can also lead to adults shaping children in their own image of childish innocence.

Romanticism played a part, and an important one in this process of softening attitudes to children and, in conjunction with a indulgent interpretation of Rousseau, it could lead to the sentimentality exhibited by the likes of Letitia Elizabeth Landon. However, eccentricities apart, Romanticism was mostly safely incorporated into a bourgeois definition of family life and its radicalness defused. But the combination of Puritan and Romantic traditions did, indeed, give rise to occasional 'weird patterns of thought', and these provide intimations of a deeper disturbance, one that would project ideas deep into the twentieth century.

Perhaps what Rousseau most significantly let loose upon the western world was a perception of the dierence between the child and the adult. Mostly we think of this in terms of opening up the scope for adult interpretations of the nature of childhood and of the child's world, but it also allowed for a child's view of adult life. Perhaps one of the most characteristic representations of the child in late twentieth-century literature and film is as a critical, occasionally cynical, observer of adult behaviour. Such a manoeuvre first appeared in the mid-nineteenth century. Cunningham, for example, notes how from the 1840s, cartoonists such as John Leech and George Cruikshank began to present the children of the streets not merely as victims but as 'a means of poking fun at the pretensions of respectability' (Cunningham, 1991: 113). Grylls also notes how fiction written for children began to acquire a similar capacity, pointing especially to a story by Anstey (like Leech associated with the magazine *Punch*), *Vice Versa*, published in 1882, in which a father and son swap physical appearances. The father then experiences life at his son's school and not only learns what it is to be a real child, but also discovers how little of the trappings and pretensions of his adult status survive his translation to childhood. Grylls calls the story a juvenile equivalent to Butler's *The Way of All Flesh* and (perhaps rather too grandly) claims it to be a 'landmark in the decline of Victorian patriarchy'. Certainly it was subversive of the didacticism and rationalism dominant earlier in the century (Grylls, 1978: 103). As a child, Anstey, it is worth noting, had read *Sandford and Merton* and his mother had attempted, as Sunday reading, to read aloud *The Fairchild Family*, but apparently the whole family laughed too much and the story had to be given up.

Another example which illustrates very graphically a tendency to present not an idealised view of the child's world, but a much starker view of its reality is Kipling's collection of school stories, *Stalky & Co.* In these stories, the bulk of which were written at the close of the nineteenth century, Kipling took the form of the boys' school story and turned it into something quite unique, distasteful to many critics but of enduring fascination. Stalky and his loyal followers M'Turk and Beetle take revenge upon fellow pupils and teachers alike in a series of fairly appalling episodes. These involve, for example, the use of the rotting corpse of a dead cat and, in a story about bullying, a degree of violence that would disturb most modern publishers of children's fiction. However, there is an adult world whose proximity casts a shadow over the antics of the boys. This is a school whose principal purpose is to prepare its pupils for future training as army ocers, a utilitarian establishment with none of the pretensions of a public school proper. Against this growing seriousness and awareness of a real world in which some of their friends will inevitably be killed, it is the teachers who appear as childish, mostly insensitive to the destiny of their pupils (Quigly, 1987).

Even more subversive of adult pretensions, of course, was Lewis Carroll (Charles Dodgson). Even as a child he used to write parodies of the didactic and moral verse with which he and his siblings were no doubt familiar. Cohen quotes one such from a family magazine the young Charles produced in 1845 when he was 13:

I have a fairy by my side
Which says I must not sleep,
When once in pain I loudly cried
It said, 'You must not weep.'

After more verses in which the fairy issues prohibitions against smiling, drinking, tasting and fighting wars, the poem concludes,

'What *may* I do?" At length I cried,
Tired of the painful task,
The fairy quietly replied,
And said, 'You must not ask.'
(quoted Cohen, 1984: 8)

Perhaps what is most significant about Carroll is not the mockery itself, but that it came from a boy and later from a man who, as Cohen argues, was a model Victorian. The distance that Carroll, through parody, puts between himself and the message does not mean that the message itself is rejected. Here, rather, are signs of an ability to be both on the inside and on the outside of what one believes. As Cohen remarks, 'these children who were taught they *mustn't* did in time go on to become adults, and carried the lesson of *mustn't* to the four corners of the earth' (1984: 8). Of course in the *Alice* books, this inside-and-outsideness is exquisitely developed, but instead of the child himself writing, Carroll has now become an adult, and uses all his adult skills to show us the absurdity of the adult world. There is no doubt that Mrs Trimmer would not have understood Carroll, would not indeed have understood how anybody could use the child in painting so bizarre, so unrealistic, so morally ambiguous a view of the world. But this serves to strengthen Grylls' argument that this major shift in perceptions of childhood is a nineteenth-century and not a twentieth-century phenomenon. It is only by turning Carroll into some kind of freak that the twentieth century can make him marginal to our perception of the Victorian world view and preserve the fiction that he is a special case only to be really understood through late twentieth-century sophistication.

The case of children's fiction is an important one in understanding the shifting nature of childhood discourses in the nineteenth century. As a vehicle for religiously inspired didacticism, children's books probably penetrated quite deeply into the consciousness of the more respectable working classes, and were clearly everyday material for the children of the growing middle classes. As has already been suggested, in children's fiction, Romanticism too did eventually find its own voice through fantasy, fleetingly in the *Phantasmion* of 1837 by Coleridge's daughter Sara, which Dennis Butts compares to Keats' *Endymion*, and more enduringly in Kingsley's *Water Babies* and George MacDonald's *At the Back of the North Wind*, both containing a combination of social realism and dream-like fantasy; and in MacDonald's stories about Curdie and Princess Irene – full of mines and goblins and an imploding city (Butts, 1995). This is not so much the Romanticism of Wordsworth, which was to be so easily domesticated, but that of Coleridge which acquired through Kingsley and MacDonald a symbolic Christianity, a belief that through the exercise of the imagination the child could reach out to and understand divine messages, that the innocence of the child, through the trials and tribulations of the story, could become something more transcendent. This moral weight, as Briggs notes, was inherited by twentieth-century writers of fantasy for children such as Tolkein and C.S. Lewis (Briggs, 1995). It is, of course, a far cry from the moral seriousness of the evangelicals, but the more perceptive amongst them (those, for example, that knew the value of *Pilgrim's Progress*) might not have been too critical. Thus, the late Victorian child was presented with a range of reflections of him or herself which would have baed children of a previous age. There was, perhaps still predominantly, the child of didactic literature, always morally suspect but with the burden of original sin lying somewhat lighter. There was the child of a more utilitarian morality, for whom good work and enterprise received their just reward. But now there was also the child of Romantic fantasy, Bunyan's Christian turned child and let loose in enchanted worlds, there to fight evil and find to find their own soul. And lastly, there was the child as critic, prober and all-too-insightful observer of adult follies. None of these figures would be unfamiliar to a late twentieth-century child, but they all owe their origins in some measure to the conflicting and often contradictory discourses that surrounded the Victorian child.

THE CHILD AS FATHER OF THE MAN

Marshall Brown has argued that Romanticism developed a historical sensibility, a curiosity about how the present relates to the past, more fully than did the Enlightenment. Not that the Enlightenment was unobservant about the irrational margins of human nature and its background of 'generative darkness', as Brown has it (Brown, 1993: 37). What Brown has in mind is Lawrence Sterne's *Tristram Shandy*, a novel of the 1760s which opens with the hero observing his own conception and bemoaning the thoughtlessness of his parents as they begat him. For as Tristram Shandy remarks in a clear parody of the opening of Locke's *Some Thoughts Concerning Education*,

> nine parts in ten of a man's sense or nonsense, his successes and miscarriages in this world depend upon [the] motions and activity [of the animal spirits transfused from father to son], and the different tracts and train you put them into, so that once they are set a-going, whether right or wrong, 'tis not a half-penny matter, – away they go cluttering like hey-go mad.
>
> (Book I, Chapter 1)

Why, asks Tristram's father at the end of the novel, 'when we go about to make and plant a man, do we put out the candle?' But in spite of Sterne's darker thoughts, the child of the Enlightenment, certainly the child we have encountered in Locke and then in Rousseau, is not encouraged to remember its origins, and certainly not encouraged to pass facetious judgements upon the manner of its own conception! However, this historical sensibility about the generative darkness from which the child comes, claims Brown, was something which Romanticism did develop. Furthermore, recollection of the past comes not only in the dreams of memory, but with the moment of awakening comes also an enhanced knowledge of the past. Thus Wordsworth, musing upon the landscape above Tintern Abbey revisited after an interval of several years, recalls how, whilst far away, the memory of the place had the power to induce

> that serene and blessed mood,
> In which the affections gently lead us on, –
> Until, the breath of this corporeal frame
> And even the motion of our human blood
> Almost suspended, we are laid asleep
> In body, and become a living soul:
> While with an eye made quiet by the power

Of harmony, and the deep power of joy,
We see into the life of things.
(1936: lines 41–9)

And the most powerful memory, for Wordsworth, is of childhood. However benign, affectionate and understanding Locke's perception of childhood might be, it is still for him a state to be abandoned, its half-knowledge rejected for the clearer light of adult perception. Hence, according to Brown, the Enlightenment 'aimed at masking and forgetting the itinerary by which it arrived at reason' whilst Romanticism aimed at 'knowing the light through knowing the dark and the present by means of the past' (Brown, 1993: 43).

At a less abstract level, the sensibility which Brown refers to can be found in Dickens. There are perhaps three aspects of his employment of the child figure which are important. First, Dickens remains a nineteenth century-folk hero, best known as the social reformer who sensitised his bourgeois readers to the plight of the poor urban child, persuading them through his writings to look at the street children with the same eyes that saw their own children. Oliver Twist, Smike and Tiny Tim have found a secure place in contemporary popular culture. Second, parenting comes under intense scrutiny in Dickens and is mostly found wanting. Parents and step-parents are cruel and too demanding of gratitude, pompous and insensitive, distant and unloving, and, like badly bought up children, overly dependent and unreasonably demanding. In *Hard Times*, first published in 1854, Dickens turns his wrath upon a father who fails to understand the nature of childhood itself. Through the disasters that befall his own children, Gradgrind learns the folly of his utilitarian approach to parenting, and has to hear the reproach of his daughter Louisa:

> How could you give me life, and take from me all the inappreciable things that raise it from the state of conscious death? Where are the graces of my soul? Where are the sentiments of my heart? What have you done, O father, what have you done with the garden that should have bloomed once, in this great wilderness here!
> (Chapter 12)

It is the very unsentimentality of the representation of the child in *Hard Times* that gives it its power and avoids the sweetness too often attached to Dickens' children. But into Louisa's mind he can put the sense of a lost childhood, of a sweetness denied. The following passage is worth quoting at length:

> Neither, as she approached her old home now, did any of the best influences of old home descend upon her. The dreams of childhood – its airy fables; its graceful, beautiful, humane, impossible adornments of the world beyond: so good to be believed in once, so good to be remembered when outgrown, for then the least among them rises to the stature of a great Charity in the heart, suffering little children to come into the midst of it, and to keep with their pure hands a garden in the stony ways of this world, wherein it were better for all children of Adam that they should oftener sun themselves, simple and trustful, and not worldly-wise – what had she to do with these? Remembrances of how she had journeyed to the little that she knew, by the enchanted roads of what she and millions of innocent creatures had hoped and imagined; of how, first coming upon Reason through the tender light of Fancy, she had seen it as a beneficent god, deferring to gods as great as itself; not a grim Idol, cruel and cold, with its victims bound hand and foot, and its big dumb shape set up with a sightless stare, never to be moved by anything but so many calculated tons of leverage – what had she to do with these? Her remembrances of home and childhood, were remembrances of the drying up of every spring and fountain in her young heart as it gushed out. The golden waters were not there. They were flowing for the fertilization of the land where grapes are gathered from thorns, and figs from thistles. 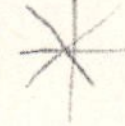
>
> (Chapter 9)

Through the excess of metaphor, it is possible to see in Dickens' assault upon utilitarian rationalism as clear an expression as one is likely to find of Romanticism's child as it developed in the nineteenth century. The child should live with nature, though nature has already become the domestic garden, and reason is not rejected but rather is to be found 'through the tender light of Fancy'. But perhaps most significantly it is the memory of childhood, again thoroughly domesticated by Dickens since childhood and home become inseparable, that is essential to the adult. Louisa cannot grow up, cannot experience adult love, because she had no childhood, no memories with which to build that 'great Charity in the heart'. And this Charity, Dickens seems to imply, is at the heart of parenting, through its capacity to 'suffer little children to come into the midst of it', a memory that allows the adult to preserve the innocence of the child.

The third sense in which Dickens' perception of childhood is important grows very much out of this centrality of childhood memory to the happiness of the adult. Andrews has cogently argued that Dickens was much exercised by the rival claims of the imagination and of reason, of fancy and of fact, as the basis for preparing the young for adult life. Dickens wrote an essay in 1860 entitled 'Mr. Barlow', in which he berated Thomas Day's Mr Barlow for being killjoy of all the natural pleasures of childhood and for inducing in the child Dickens a sense of guilt at the enjoyment of these pleasures. Day's rationalism becomes conflated with the evangelicism of Mrs Trimmer as part of a crusade to kill the very essence of childhood. In retreat before this onslaught, Dickens says he took 'refuge in the caves of ignorance, wherein I have resided ever since, and which are still my private address' (quoted Andrews, 1994: 39). Especially critical for Dickens as a novelist, claims Andrews, is that he strove to preserve in maturity the childhood capacity to fuse imagination and reality. In many ways this is similar to Wordsworth's aspirations, a desire as Coleridge expressed it

> To carry on the feelings of childhood into the powers of manhood, to combine the child's sense of wonder and novelty with the appearances which every day for perhaps forty years had rendered familiar.
>
> (quoted Andrews, 1994: 25)

However, Andrews detects a shift away from the early Romantics in that Dickens felt more trapped by the demands made of maturity in the mid-nineteenth century, by the growing separation of the cultural worlds of the child and adult that became increasingly difficult to bridge. By the end of the century, claims Coveney, the task for some, like Sir James Barrie with *Peter Pan*, had become impossible, but for Dickens there could and should be a 'mutually tolerant partnership', as Andrews puts it, if not a fusion between the child and the adult (Coveney, 1967; Andrews, 1994). This leaves childhood as a kind of counterculture which can help preserve the grown-up child in each of us, an adult 'whose personality, the interior child and interior grown-up are endlessly reconstituting' (Andrews, 1994: 174).

It is appropriate to end this discussion of Romanticism and the child by returning to Wordsworth, but specifically to a study that searches for the contemporary significance of Wordsworth. Antony Easthope finds in the poetry of this patriarch of the Romantic movement the origins of a contemporary narcissism, the origins of a resonance that reaches down from Romanticism right through to

Frank Sinatra's assurance that since, whatever he did he did it his way, there could be few regrets. As Easthope puts it,

> What Wordsworth's poetry so vividly exemplifies is the self's struggle to extricate itself from the defiles of the Other – to find a version of language which seems to belong only to itself, to address an Other almost identical with itself, to find itself reflected in an Other as much like itself as possible, to admit loss as a means of recuperating it, and so on and so on, at all events to be an 'I am' and not 'I will have been'.
>
> (Easthope, 1993: 128)

Easthope explores the poetry of Wordsworth through the post-structuralist psychoanalysis of Lacan. For Lacan, the baby has to leave the realm of the 'real', a place of unity and complete fulfilment in the womb of the mother, and to find an identity, or rather some identification, away from the mother. In the image of itself in the mirror the child sees or thinks it sees itself, but what it really sees is an image, more co-ordinated, more whole than the fragmented creature that looks, in fact an illusion. From this first illusion, the infant moves on to enter the world of language, a world of signs and meanings which existed prior to the child's own being and which position it and provide an illusory identity deriving, not from some inner core of the child's being, but from an already structured realm of symbolic meanings existing outside the child. As a word or a symbol in language acquires its meaning, not from any intrinsic quality, but simply because it is different from and therefore distinguishable from another word or symbol, so the identity of the child is defined in relation to others. But the human infant forever lives in search of that moment of fullness in the womb, in search of the wholeness of the image in the mirror and in search of the language that will define the self without reference to another. The cry of the baby is first a need for food and then a demand for love, and finally an expression of desire that can never find fulfilment.

'Why does the child turn round to look at the Other?', asks Madan Sarup. The answer is that, 'The Other warrants the existence of the child, certifies the dierence between self and other. . . . In a way the Other is the real witness and guarantor of the subject's existence' (Sarup, 1992: 64, 98). Terry Eagleton perhaps best summarises this mysterious 'Other':

> Language, the unconscious, the parents, the symbolic order: these

terms in Lacan are not exactly synonymous, but they are intimately allied. They are sometimes spoken of by him as the 'Other' – as that which like language is always anterior to us and will always escape us, that which brought us into being as subjects in the first place but which will always outrun our grasp . . . for Lacan our unconscious desire is directed towards this Other, in the shape of some ultimately gratifying reality which we can never have; but it is also true for Lacan that our desire is in some way always *received* from the Other too. We desire what others – our parents for instance – unconsciously desire for us; and desire can only happen because we are caught up in linguistic, sexual and social relations – the whole field of the 'Other' – which generate it.

(Eagleton, 1983: 174)

We have already noted in the previous chapter Wordsworth's dismay at the coming of mass society; Easthope identifies this as at the heart of the Romantic ideology. In Lacanian terms the sense of lack that generates desire is at once more obvious and more difficult to fill, hence 'the subject works harder to imagine its way into an autonomous and meaningful identity for itself' (Easthope, 1993: 21). For Wordsworth this becomes the poet's search for an identity constructed by the imagination. Hence:

My heart leaps up when I behold
A rainbow in the sky:
So was it when I first began:
So is it now I am a man:
So let it be when I grow old,
Or let me die!
The Child is father of the Man:
And I could wish my days to be
Bound each to each by natural piety.

This is Easthope's commentary:

No other work in the *oeuvre* so perfectly epitomises so many Wordsworthian themes and effects. It expresses a simple wish that the self continue as a single identity from the past, across the present and into the future so that each moment of time could make up a kind of personal time, in which the days of the calendar and habitual chronology should be 'my days' (not someone else's) 'bound' (not just linked) by a natural unity so that, in reverse of the usual paternal origin, the experience of the child founds that of the

> adult man, this unfathered boy somehow originating himself, without dad.
>
> (Easthope, 1993: 34)

But this is impossible, since no identity can be constructed without a pre-existing language, a parent, an Other. It is through the sense of difference from the Other, not in the sense of unity with the self, that identity is formed. Wordsworth's attempt to solve the impossible is through autobiography, by making his own childhood self the Other. Thus that moment of awakening in 'Tintern Abbey' to which Marshall Brown referred, that moment when 'we are laid asleep/In body, and become a living soul', is one that guarantees the continuity and transcendence of individual identity. And whilst Tristram Shandy saw destiny in the manner of his own conception, Romanticism turns autobiography into an affirmation of the inevitable by 're-imagining the traces of memories' (ibid.: 89).

For Easthope, then, Romanticism is responsible for an attempt to deny the social, determined nature of our identity, a denial that he believes can be heard time and again in popular song in the late twentieth century, an expression of the 'commonality of our privacy', of the inescapable fact that 'what I most share with others is the desire to be dierent from them' (ibid.: 126). Through Romanticism there enters into western societies one of the central tensions that inhabits contemporary child-rearing; the desire to sponsor individualism, to create in the growing child a sense of a unique autobiography with its own unique store of memories; and at the same time a desire to stay within the bounds of normality, to live up to the standards of a defining and repressive Other. Romanticism, of course, was not alone responsible for this; the connection between modernity and individualism is an often retold tale. Nevertheless in Easthope's reading of Wordsworth one can see the desire, the yearning and the sense of loss that so often in the nineteenth and twentieth centuries has found a focus in childhood. The movement beyond Rousseau's cool-headed concern for the integrity of the child is striking, and, before him, Locke's aim was for an individual whose sense of reason would be uncluttered by convention and tradition, not for the 'self-creating, self-regarding identity' of Wordsworth (Langbaum, quoted ibid.: 127).

Perhaps of most significance is the way in which Romanticism oered a means of social criticism, a stick with which to beat the hegemony of the evangelical rationalism. Flaunting the virtues of imagination, flirting with the child of nature in its many guises, elevating motherhood to an almost mystical state and, perhaps most eectively, mocking religious didacticism as antithetical to the very nature of childhood, the Romantics and their heirs provided a challenge which caught the imagination. On the one hand it gave a special meaning to those social reformers who campaigned on behalf of children, since the tribe of children could be used, en masse as it were, to force government to acknowledge the social consequence of industrialisation and rapid urbanisation. On the other hand, the child gave a special meaning and purpose to the bourgeois home and garden, providing a focus for the cult of domesticity and a justification as clear as that of the Puritans for a strictly gendered division of labour.

Probably Romanticism was always a countercultural movement and never an orthodoxy; when it came to practicalities it was (as an eighteenth-century aristocratic lady once described Rousseau's proposals) not practical but 'immensely pretty' (Trumbach, 1978). Whether its legacy for the late twentieth century is to be regarded in a positive or negative light is very dicult to answer, but two points should, perhaps, be stressed. One is the clearly negative eect Romanticism had upon Puritan and evangelical conceptions of child-rearing, and specifically upon the divinely delegated authority of parents. Many other factors, for good or bad, have eroded parental authority, but there is a case to be made for Grylls' argument that Romanticism's assault upon the evangelicals was a decisive turning point.

The second point has more to do with the representation of childhood. The decline into sentimentality, which Coveney noted, has much to do with this problem of representation, and on a broader front Easthope too refers to the rhetoric of the imagination and pathos as key aspects of Romantic expression which do not have wholly positive consequences. There is much to be said for the view that one of the most significant eects of Romanticism upon childhood was to expose the problematic nature of the representation of childhood. The translation of the Romantic child from his origins as a noble savage to the landscapes of northern England and from thence to the urban ghettoes of the growing cities and to the suburban gardens of the bourgeoisie, gave rise to a rhetoric of imagination and pathos that has been all too briefly sketched here. Furthermore the child was to be found in new forms of representation; in popular poetry and song for the middle classes, as cartoon figure and perhaps most significantly as the central character in poetry and stories designed for the child's own consumption. This fictional representation of the child is of a richness and variety that had never previously existed, and it is here as much as anywhere that the vitality of Romanticism is to be found and is carried forward to the mass media and popular cultural forms of the twentieth century. What of course matters most about this is that these are not merely representations *of* children, but representations *to* children, manifestations of the Other which so powerfully shape the narrative of the self through autobiography.

Chapter 6

The child of the Victorians

Gender and sexuality in childhood

> A Child of Thirteen Bought for £5
>
> At the beginning of this Derby week, a woman, an old hand in the work of procuration, entered a brothel in _____st. M_______, kept by an old acquaintance, and opened negotiations for the purchase of a maid. One of the women who lodged in the house had a sister as yet untouched. Her mother was far away, her father was dead. The child was living in the house, and in all probability would be seduced and follow the profession of her elder sister. The child was between thirteen and fourteen, and after some bargaining it was agreed that she should be handed over to the procuress for the sum of £5.
>
> *Pall Mall Gazette*, 1885

It is perhaps with respect to the Victorians' view of childhood sexuality that contemporary wisdom is most inclined to see a confusion of the Romantic and the Puritan view of the child. On the one hand there is no doubting the sensuality that Lewis Carroll, for example, found in the image of the young girl, most obviously in the nude photographs which are difficult for the late twentieth-century mind to see except as sexualised images. On the other hand, towards the end of the century, some more extreme members of the Social Purity movement, in the wake of a moral panic about the supposed extent of child prostitution, sought to delay the sexual independence of girls until they were 21. Romanticism led to an aesthetic that adored the purity of the young child's unclothed form, but in the hands of a 'Puritan' morality it could also lead to something prudish and suffocating, the stereotype of Victorian repressive stuffiness. As with Puritanism itself, we are faced here with the rewriting of history and, in particular, with the way in which the twentieth century has interpreted Victorian sexual behaviour and attitudes.

Mason has argued that we have a special relationship to the Victorians. The very term 'Victorian' has far more emotional connotative power than ever 'Tudor' or 'Georgian' could now muster. Even at the end of the twentieth century, it still seems to be the first 'historical' period we meet going backwards. 'Before the turn of the century', says Mason, 'lies the other, the irrevocable, the strange – human beings who are not like us and who are sundered from us by the power of the historical processes' (Mason, 1994a: 1). And yet, he claims, because they are the first such age they awaken in us feelings of hostility as well as of nostalgia and admiration, producing a mix which is quite distinctive in our historical perceptions. Furthermore, given the twentieth century preoccupation with sexual liberation and tolerance, and a steady pressure which strives to break down sexual rules and to speak publicly about what was previously private, it is not surprising that we use Victorian sexual moralism as a focus for our hostility. It may also be the case that the Victorians themselves, continuing a trend evident in the eighteenth century, did in fact increasingly organise morality around sexual behaviour and attitudes, thus narrowing the scope of virtue to cover only sexual chastity (Watt, 1957; Weeks, 1981: 23; Spilka, 1984).

It is not surprising, either, that the epithet 'Puritan' should be applied to Victorian sexual behaviour and attitudes, and that, since the work of writers like Marcus and Pearsall on Victorian pornography and feminist critiques of the 'double-standard' of sexual behaviour, Victorian puritanism has become associated with hypocrisy (Marcus, 1967; Pearsall, 1983; Vicinus, 1972, 1980). In any case there were enough Victorians prepared to describe the activities and attitudes of their fellows as 'Puritan'. In the debates over the Contagious Diseases Acts, for example, the *Saturday Review*, a journal frequently critical of Victorian sentimentality and religiosity, accused those sectarian groups who wanted greater police efforts against prostitution of 'Puritanic prudery', and W.R. Greg musing upon the possibility of men as well as women being able to subdue sexual desire before marriage was fearful of sounding 'puritanic or Quixotic' (Mason, 1994b: 97). Even so, there is a shift in emphasis from the Victorians own critique of prudishness to that of the latter half of the twentieth century. Flaunting its own imagined sexual liberation, the twentieth-century mind dismisses the Victorians as sexually repressed: according to Kincaid, our grandfathers 'called the Victorians "prudish", whilst we call them "repressed"' (Kincaid, 1992: 33). The difference, for Kincaid, lies in the totality of our explanation. Whilst 'prudishness' merely suggests what is being avoided, a fear of the erotic which is known to exist but cannot be talked about, 'repression' (to an age which has consumed, digested and largely evacuated Freud) is simply a smug term of total and undeniable explanation. The Victorians were repressed; repression is bad; that is all we need to know.

In fact, of course, since Foucault, our smugness has had to be rethought, and 'prudish' seems once again a not inappropriate term to describe a society in which sex, even when unspoken, was at the centre of discourse. Sex, according to Foucault, was at the heart of an exercise of power concerned not to repress (which would render power fragile), but rather to discipline the body and make sex the subject of policy; that is to say, in need of policing (Foucault, 1984; Donzelot, 1980). Thus sexuality, increasingly, became from the end of the eighteenth century, 'an especially dense transfer point for relations of power: between men and women, young people and old people, parents and offspring, teachers and students, priests and laity, and administration and a population' (Foucault, 1984: 103). However, if it is all as serious as this, then 'prudish', however well it conveys a sense of barely concealed curiosity, will not really do. In any case prudishness itself was an adjective thrown around the western world with abandon in the nineteenth century. It was employed, for example, by the French against the English, and by the English against the Americans. Only a few of the more common jibes about chicken 'bosoms' and covered furniture legs seem to stand up to historical scrutiny as evidence of widespread behaviour (Mason, 1994a: 128). The message that should be taken from Foucault is not only that the repressive hypothesis needs to be rethought, but also that through the discourses on sexuality we have the opportunity to glimpse the heart of human relationships in the Victorian era, not least those between parents and children and more broadly between the adult and the child.

NINETEENTH-CENTURY ANTI-SENSUALISM

However, even if the general repressive hypothesis has been successfully challenged, the link between religion and sexual behaviour is still presumed to be strong. Rather as the *Saturday Review* used to do in the nineteenth century, there is still a tendency in the twentieth century to regard not only 'Puritan' but also Catholic religious practice as antithetical to enlightened sex education. Twentieth-century novels such as Jeanette Winterson's *Oranges Are Not the Only Fruit* or Berlie Doherty's *Requiem* tend to confirm the myth of religion as a repressive force which distorts normal sexual development. A recent challenge to the presumed connection between repressive attitudes to sex and religious belief has come from Mason's research into nineteenth-century sexual behaviour and attitudes. There was indeed, argues Mason, a strong anti-sensual tradition from the late eighteenth century right through to the end of the nineteenth, but it was a progressive strand of thought which had its origins in the Enlightenment belief in the superiority of reason over emotion. Religion, however, especially amongst dissenting and non-conformist groups, was much more ambiguous in its attitude to sensuality and eroticism throughout most of the nineteenth century. On the one hand, evangelicism could on occasion ally itself with progressive thought and give weight to anti-sensualism, but on the other hand religious fervour was never far away from eroticism. Though Mason confirms the sobriety of most religious sects, he does note that accusing fingers were pointed, for example, at the sensuality and sexual imagery of some Methodist devotional material. In addition, of course, there were a few sects, as there had been in the mid-seventeenth century, for whom sexuality became a central feature. Mason concludes that, in general, the common charge of antinomianism and sexual licence amongst the religious sects was an unfounded slur, but nor does he find, except amongst the more extreme Social Purity advocates of the late nineteenth and early twentieth centuries, a sexually repressive morality (Mason 1994a, b).

One important source for the anti-sensual tradition that Mason identifies is Rousseau's *Emile*, 'an endocrine gland in the system of English nineteenth-century anti-sensualism' (Mason, 1994b: 15). Whilst, for Rousseau, reason needs the spur of feeling and remains arid without it, sexual desire is not a physical need, it is not a 'true need'. It is, he claims, imagination that wakens the senses; hence they are culturally not biologically shaped. The savage 'raised in a desert, without books, without instruction, without women, would die there a virgin at whatever age he had reached' (Rousseau, 1979: 333). Emile himself is urged to a degree of asceticism, not in order to emulate the savage in the desert, but to make the joys of marital love all the sweeter. Rousseau does, however, enter a rather sour note by suggesting that the anticipation is better than reality ever can be. In one sense, it is all of a piece. Society which corrupts the mind corrupts also the emotions and even distorts human instincts. It is Rousseau's belief in the cultural origins of sexuality that, according to Mason, is reflected in nineteenth-century anti-sensualism. Rousseau did give rise directly to at least one early nineteenth-century attempt to advocate scientific sex education as an antidote to the unbridled imagination (that of Thomas Beddoes who married into the Edgeworth family), but his influence is generally more diffuse, lending intellectual weight to a more general movement (Mason, 1994b).

It is wrong, argues Mason, to associate this anti-sensual tradition very closely with religion. Its origins in the Enlightenment belief in rationality make it, for much of the nineteenth century, a progressive movement. It is more closely associated with nineteenth-century environmentalism, a progressive belief that behaviour is affected by circumstance rather than nature. Much religiously motivated social reform was influenced by environmentalism too, but this was always at odds with a continuing belief in original sin. The tension emerged, for example, in conflicting views of the origins and consequences of prostitution. A more religious, more sensualist view, saw in prostitution a re-enactment of the Fall, and saw the possibility of redemption only through penance and ritual humiliation. To the more 'rational' Victorian, prostitution was a response to economic circumstance, a stage of life that was as likely to end with marriage as with anything more dramatic. And when mixed with feminism, prostitution could become not only economically rational, but a defensible manifestation of female independence. When, as in the figure of the campaigning Josephine Butler, evangelicism, environmentalism and feminism combined, the mixture could be both powerful and ambiguous (Mason, 1994b).

It is possible, of course, to see in the religious response to prostitution a fear of the sensual and a desire to repress it, and it is this that several commentators have seen emerging in the Social Purity movement of the late nineteenth century. Through campaigns against prostitution, including child prostitution, against homosexuality and masturbation, against lax aristocratic morals in particular and the double standard of sexual morality in general, the Social Purity movement exerted considerable influence through the last years of Victoria's reign and on into the Edwardian era. But even here religious anti-sensualism found occasional support from more radical and rationalist movements. For the most part middle class and nonconformist in its origins, the Social Purity movement, on occasions such as the campaign against child prostitution, found unlikely support from feminists, liberal lawyers, socialists and Anglican bishops. Clearly, too, in its attack upon upper class morality, it struck a chord amongst sections of the working class. It was 'Puritan' in its outlook, taking the search for purity from its sixteenth- and seventeenth-century forebears, but its focus was almost exclusively on sexual behaviour (Weeks, 1981; Mason, 1994a, b; Walkowitz, 1980, 1982; Jeffreys, 1985). The general tenor of their campaigns did, however, also spill over into propaganda about baby care and child-rearing in general, though often with sexual overtones. Walkowitz, for example, suggests that,

> The prescriptive literature distributed by social purity groups also seems to have influenced the child-rearing practices of the time. Edwardian working-class parents were notable for their strict schedules, puritanical treatment of masturbation, and for the severe restrictions they placed on their teenage daughter's social and sexual behaviour.
>
> (Walkowitz, 1982: 86)

It is, therefore, only at the end of the Victorian period that a sexually repressive Puritanism can be found. Too often, perhaps, the broad moral thrust of dissenting and evangelical movements from the early nineteenth century has been collapsed into the preoccupations of late Victorian Social Purity movements with their much narrower sexual focus. As a consequence the complexities of much nineteenth-century discourse on sexuality have been ignored and the contradictions crudely explained away as a mixture of repressive tendencies and gross hypocrisy.

THE SEXUALITY OF THE CHILD

For Foucault, the history of sexuality in the west since the seventeenth century is a long process of 'turning sex into discourse', of shaping accounts which describe, define and indeed create new areas of sexuality, which persuade us to confess, to tell, or to transform desire into religious ecstasy and perhaps even into rational endeavour. 'An immense verbosity is what our civilization has required and organised', says Foucault (1984: 33). In this grand scheme of things, 'the reticences of "Victorian puritanism" ' are to be viewed as an historical accident, or 'at any rate . . . a digression, a refinement, a tactical diversion in the great process of transforming sex into discourse' (ibid.: 22). One of the most important of these emerging discourses was concerned with the sexuality of children. The freedom of language between children and adults as evinced, for example, at the beginning of the seventeenth century in the relations between the little Louis XIII and his father, mother and servants was gradually restricted (Ariès, 1973: 98). This, claims Foucault, was not 'a plain and simple imposition of silence', it was part of the process of turning sex into discourse. It was not that less was said, but that it was said in a different way. And silence itself,

> the things one declines to say, or is forbidden to name, the discretion that is required between different speakers – is less the absolute limit of discourse, the other side from which it is separated by a strict boundary, than an element that functions alongside the things said, with them and in relation to them within over-all strategies.
>
> (Foucault, 1984: 27)

Discourses, for Foucault, are strategies for the exercise of power. In relation to childhood, they define not only, for children themselves, the scope and limitations of childhood, but also define the relationship of others to children. Hence discourses on sexuality seek to delineate and control not only the nature of sexual desire in children, but also to define adult love towards children and, indeed, the love of children for each other. For example, the wish to define children as asexual, or at least in a state of sexual latency, produced in the nineteenth and early twentieth centuries a flood of measures to control masturbation (Neuman, 1974). In Foucault's terms, masturbation was driven into hiding – into silence as it were – and then traps were set, surveillance increased, and parents alerted by prognostications of dire consequences if they failed in their vigilance. But discourses about sexuality define adult relationships to children as well and devise strategies accordingly. For example, in the Edwardian period, it was important to warn against governesses who taught their charges to masturbate; between the wars, to warn against over-loving mothers who over-excited their offspring, in the late twentieth century against potential paedophiles (Stainton Rogers, 1992: 170; Beekman, 1978; Kincaid, 1992).

There is a danger in using Foucault's concept of discourses that we make them appear too tidy, too intellectually coherent and also that we neglect the resistance that is inherent in any power struggle. In looking at Victorian discourses on childhood sexuality, it is important to look at the way in which contradictions and ambiguities came to the surface. As Kincaid has pointed out these are of central importance not only in understanding the Victorians, but also in understanding the extent and depth of the legacy they have left to the twentieth century. Perhaps, after all, one of the most important aspects of Foucault's intervention into discussion of the history of sexuality was to connect us very firmly to the Victorians, rather than to separate us from them.

Central to discourses upon childhood sexuality is a denial of that sexuality, but one of the possible consequences of that denial is that childhood is eroticised. To stress the purity, innocence and beauty of childhood is, as Kincaid puts it, to 'create a subversive echo: experience, corruption, eroticism' (Kincaid, 1992: 5). As Pattison has shown, this contradiction is, in terms of literary expression, a very old one, glimpsed even in classical times (Pattison, 1978). Closer to home, Pattison finds similar sentiments in the seventeenth-century Puritan poet Andrew Marvell, who gazing upon a little girl, 'T.C.', as she plays amongst the flowers, sees simplicity and harmony with nature. But Marvell feels also the threat of her latent sexual power: 'Let me be laid', he says, 'Where I may see thy Glories from some shade.' He longs for her to use her power as child of nature to remove the thorns from the Rose, but also to grant the Violets a longer life so that their moment of bloom is not so brief. But most important of all, he warns his little T.C. to pick only the fully grown flowers and not the buds,

> Lest Flora angry at thy crime,
> To kill her Infants in their prime,
> Do quickly make th 'Example Yours;
> And, ere we see,
> Nip in the blossome all our hopes and Thee.
> (Picture of Little T.C. in a Prospect of Flowers, 1681)

Thus childhood sexuality, present only in the child's innocent simplicity, threatens the poet's peace and disturbs his equanimity. But at the same time he becomes fearful of its fragility, its all too brief moment of bloom. In this anticipatory moment, before full female sexuality, both the Rose with its power to wound and the Violet with its fragile beauty are held seemingly in the power of the child herself. Thus Marvell weaves around the little girl a fantasy of both innocence and potency which leaves him fearful both of her power and of the fragile nature of that power.

There is nothing strange, argues Kincaid, about the way in which adults see the beauty of children. 'I can see and feel', he writes, 'that the enticing images of purity and almost formless innocence are fulfilled not simply in heaven, the virgin and Ivory soap but in the child; I do not find the appeal of Shirley Temple or Freddie Bartholemew or Brooke Shields or Rick Schroeder a mystery' (Kincaid, 1992: 10). There is then a line of beautiful children that goes from Horace's Lalage, through Marvell's T.C., Wordsworth's Lucy, Carroll's Alice Liddell, Hodgson Burnett's Lord Fauntleroy and on to the child stars of the film industry. For Kincaid, what is critical about all such children is the absence which we, as adults, fill:

> This purity, this harmlessness is presented as complete vacancy; the absence of harmfulness amounts, in fact, to nothing at all, a blank image waiting to be formed.... Purity it turns out, provided just the opening a sexualising tendency requires; it is the necessary condition for the erotic operations our cultures have made central.
> (Kincaid, 1992: 13)

Childhood sexuality, like beauty, lies in the eye of the poet, the writer, the film-maker and finally in that of the beholder.

Gender and childhood: boys

It is perhaps inevitable that discussions of gender and sexuality in childhood focus primarily upon girls, though innocence and beauty are by no means confined to them. It is important, nevertheless, to make a short excursion into the way boys were perceived during the course of the nineteenth century. The traditional view of the Victorian male child tends again to be drawn from the end of the Victorian era, when the very popular adventure stories of G.A. Henty, filled with lads not over-endowed intellectually but full of 'pluck', were much in vogue. The whole perception is overlaid with a sense of the overwhelming importance of Empire. The boys of Kipling's *Stalky and Co.*, for example, are certainly being educated to defend the Empire, and his most famous poem 'If' is frequently taken as a statement of the qualities required of a true British male. But, whilst Henty may be relatively straightforward, Kipling's boys are altogether more thoughtful, more aware of the complexities of life and, indeed, of the value of forms of cultural expression far removed from the military. Beetle, after all, based upon Kipling himself, knows that he will never be a soldier and that the pen, not the sword, is his medium. Equally the poem, 'If', in spite of its final address – 'Yours is the Earth and everything that's in it,/ And – which is more – you'll be a Man, my son!' – is more introverted than its reputation would imply. Kipling himself was clearly embarrassed by the reputation the poem quickly earned and found a context for it in *Rewards and Fairies*, a series of far from imperialistic, magical tales of British history told to a little boy and girl, Dan and Una, deep in the Sussex countryside. Recent research has done much to explore the richness of nineteenth-century notions of masculinity and the critical reappraisal of Kipling's writings for children is but one small step on the way (Mangan and Walvin, 1987; Quigly, 1987; Mackenzie, 1993).

It is clear, however, that two images of the ideal boy existed at the end of the nineteenth century. One, certainly, was the action-man hero, whether found in its simple form as one of Henty's boys, or in Kipling's more complex characterisations. But the other model is to be found in Frances Hodgson Burnett's *Little Lord Fauntleroy*, American of course in origin, but clearly familiar and attractive to a British readership. His beauty (which we, but not the Victorians, label feminine) is combined with a sensitivity and intelligence which appears to be a far cry from the imperialistic lads of the late nineteenth-century adventure story. Whilst the adventure stories probably had a greater social reach than did Hodgson Burnett's tale, there were many amongst the middle classes who dressed their children like Cedric Erroll, including the parents of A.A. Milne.

Mangan and Walvin point to a change that overcame the concept of 'manliness' in the latter part of the century:

> To the early Victorian [manliness] represented a concern with a successful transition from Christian immaturity to maturity, demonstrated by earnestness, selflessness and integrity; to the late Victorian it stood for neo-Spartan virility as exemplified by stoicism, hardiness and endurance.
>
> (Mangan and Walvin, 1987: 1)

But it may well also be that there was a shift, in relation to children, away from a more androgynous conception of childhood to one which was more sharply gendered. Claudia Nelson (1989) has begun to explore the origins of these shifting images of masculinity, arguing that the power of the late Victorian stereotype has 'over-powered earlier versions of the Victorian boyish ideal'. She argues that, as the growth of evolutionary, biological discourses in the late nineteenth century displaced religious explanations of human behaviour, so an androgynous conception of the child was gradually replaced with a gendered one. This change was reflected most clearly perhaps in the growth of a gendered children's literature. In the rational and evangelical traditions of the early nineteenth century, for example in Maria Edgeworth or Mrs Sherwood, gender is not an issue; enterprise, industry and morality know of no gender distinctions. But beyond that, suggests Nelson, there is a connection made between the feminine, the asexual, the pure and the Godly. We have noted earlier in this book that the Puritans found in God both male and female characteristics, and Nelson observes that the Victorians found in the figure of Christ a chastity and a tenderness, a purity and love which they could describe as 'manly'. Hence, in Nelson's key example, Hughes' *Tom Brown's Schooldays*, Tom, at Rugby School under the watchful eye of Dr Arnold, has to learn these same Christian virtues. These he learns partly through the example of the delicate Arthur, but also through his own experience, as he has to take care of Arthur and watch over him with an almost motherly devotion. Dr Arnold, himself playing the part of the perfect parent, steers Tom to a state of manliness, a state, as Nelson puts it, when 'the boy has become a real man, gentle, pious, humble, obedient, disciplined and ready to shed a tear on affecting occasions'. The 'manly' boy of the mid-Victorian period was more likely to be found in or by the sickbed than on the playing field (Nelson, 1989: 526, 538).

The moral and spiritual qualities of the mid-century ideal boy could also draw strength from the belief in women as, by nature, less motivated by sexual feelings than men. In their state of unawakened sexuality, chaste women and all children shared a common nature. Mason, and also Kincaid, have recently questioned how generally this view of female sexuality was actually held, but it certainly was voiced and, even if it was an extreme view, it is still significant in discussions of the ideal (Mason, 1994a; Kincaid, 1992: 163). It may well be that those who voiced such a view, even when claiming medical backing, were expressing an ideal, a specific instance of the more general anti-sensual tradition with particular relevance to women and children. From their asexuality women derived their moral superiority, and children too could acquire another tint to their innocence – a superior perception and moral instinct. We have noted in a previous chapter that Dr Arnold was uncertain as to how much in the way of Christian behaviour could be expected from the growing boy. But the ideal of manliness that Arnold was so influential in advancing could draw upon several sources. There was the Christian tradition of spirituality, unloved by the evangelicals perhaps, but gaining a stronger foothold in Victorian Anglicanism. And then there were those cultural developments in the domestic role of women which had been elaborated in the early nineteenth century and the growing association of the Romantic innocence of the child with the purity of women. The 'manly' boy was wrapped around by both feminine and Romantic associations in a manner difficult for the twentieth-century mind to appreciate.

There were also more practical consequences to this. Since boys could, as it were, join girls within the category of childhood this served to emphasise the asexuality of both boys and girls. Whilst children's literature seemed merely gender blind, several commentators have pointed out that mid-nineteenth century child-rearing and sex manuals more actively encouraged an androgynous approach to children and saw little purpose in emphasising gender (Gorham, 1982; Nelson, 1989; Kincaid, 1992). If, for boys as well as girls, sexuality was dormant until awakened, the educational project could be to keep them away from situations that might awaken any sense of their own sexuality; to bring them up, as W.R. Greg suggested, with 'the same watchful attention to purity' that marked the education of girls (quoted Nelson, 1989: 532). Puritan theology, however, was still strong enough to suggest that all children would be prey to temptations, and particularly nasty temptations could be found in dormant sexuality. It is, therefore, not surprising that issues like masturbation rose to the surface as a particularly offensive childhood sin. In mid-century it was associated not only with the causes of physical and mental illness but also with spiritual loss, with the defilement of childhood's purity and with a debilitating moral egotism. Only later, for boys specifically, was masturbation more closely associated with effeminacy and homosexuality.

It is, in fact, difficult to know to what extent this approval of androgyny was the product of gender blindness, common sense or a more positive attempt to feminise boys, but there would seem to be traces of all these elements. Nevertheless Nelson has made a good case for there being a strong element of the last in the minds of at least some mid-Victorians and it is interesting to observe Romanticism's notions of innocence and purity combining with the bourgeois perceptions of the moral superiority of women and a sexology that desexualised women, to provide evangelicism with a programme of moral and spiritual training for boys. Nelson cites one American doctor, George Napheys, who caught this turmoil of ideas perfectly when he said 'it is far more accurate to say the child is mother to the woman than father to the man' (quoted Nelson, 1989: 533).

It is not a question of writing gender out of the discussion, but rather of not assuming a sharp and stereotypical gender division. But nor should it be assumed that this 'manly' child was merely a *feminised* Victorian boy. Even Little Lord Fauntleroy, late as he is in the century, is as much *sui generis*, a child of his time, as is one of Henty's heroes. Each refers to competing and intertwining Victorian discourses on gender, sexuality and childhood, embodying different conceptions of manliness and of religion, of anti-sensualism (should the sublimation of desire be achieved through mental or physical effort?), and of dependence and independence. Lord Fauntleroy's beauty is physical, but he also has spiritual, moral, and even rational qualities in his perception of adult folly. His charm is also, no doubt, heightened by his loyalty and devotion to his mother. Nevertheless, it is worth remembering that a Henty hero (Cuthbert of *Winning His Spurs* will serve as an example) also possesses a not overly masculine physical attractiveness, including the curls:

> A casual observer glancing at his curling hair and bright open face, as also at the fashion of his dress, would at one have assigned to him a purely Saxon origin; but a keener eye would have detected signs that Norman blood ran also in his veins, for his figure was lither and lighter, his features more straightly and shapely cut than was common among Saxons. His dress consisted of a tight-fitting jerkin, descending nearly to his knees.
>
> (Chapter 1)

Cuthbert, however, proceeds not by innocently probing questions and moral example, as does Lord Fauntleroy, but by direct, physical action made possible by his evident but unobtrusive athleticism. He has (unusually we are told) 'a certain amount of book learning' but it 'had not been acquired so cheerfully or willingly as the skill at arms' and,

> To do Cuthbert justice, he had protested with all his might against the proposition of Father Francis to his mother to teach him some clerkly knowledge.
>
> (Chapter 5)

In spite of being fatherless like Fauntleroy, Cuthbert is far from being dependent upon his mother, winning her permission to go to the crusades. Upon parting, his mother and the Earl's little daughter (destined, of course, to be Cuthbert's wife at the end of the tale) are allowed to cry copiously, but Henty allows to Cuthbert 'only the hard task to prevent tears filling his eyes'. Religion, Henty tells us, is not the primary motive of the crusades, rather it is the warlike nature of a people seeking escape from the monotony of castle and hut. Jeffrey Richards has made a good case for regarding Henty as a firm disciple of Samuel Smiles, author of *Self-Help* and, to twentieth-century ears, one of the most masculine of Victorian writers. Richards suggests that titles like *Winning His Spurs* could almost be a chapter heading from Smiles' writings (Richards, 1982: 54). But the enterprising child is, as we have seen, at least as old as Maria Edgeworth when gender was irrelevant; it took almost a hundred years for enterprise to become, at least for children, a purely masculine quality.

The older view of 'manliness', of Christian 'humanliness', may have begun to lose some of its credibility in the closing decades of the nineteenth century. According to Nelson, under the general influence of evolutionary theories (though one cannot help noting the natural savage again, dressed in the clothes of recapitulation theory), there emerged the image of the natural boy, at home rather than at odds with his physicality, unencumbered by spirituality and anxious, above all, to avoid the charge of effeminacy. These were Henty's boys, and harbingers of the stereotype of the twentieth-century public schoolboy, from Frank Richards' Harry Wharton to Enid Blyton's Julian and C.S. Lewis's High King Peter (Richards, 1988). These are youths of integrity and honesty no doubt, but above all they are committed to quick decision making and to action; not to reflection, or introverted moral anxiety.

There is clearly a process of gendering the child taking place during the Victorian era which deserves much fuller examination, particularly in relation to boys, and Nelson may well be right in arguing that there was a general movement away from mid-century androgyny to a more gendered conception of childhood in the late nineteenth century. One further point, however, needs to be made before leaving this issue. Kincaid has argued that it is important to explore the continuing way in which childhood qualities, not least those of eroticism and latent sexuality, override gender distinctions. When the image of the child is projected into its future, and when that future is viewed more in secular than religious terms, then gender becomes increasingly important, but when the image dwells upon the quality of the child itself the question of gender recedes into the background. Kincaid, for example, in his discussion of paedophilia, argues in relation to both the Victorians and the twentieth century that the child who is the object of paedophilia, and more generally the eroticised child of the adult imagination, is genderless. Not only does he point out that the naked bottom of the child, that ubiquitous aspect of nineteenth-century child pornography, is genderless, but he argues also that in the eroticised child of mainstream entertainment in the twentieth century, gender differences are obscured:

> these children pay little explicit attention to their bodies, are so far from being vain that they are very nearly unaware that we are watching and certainly don't notice if a shirttail is out, some underwear provocatively flashing, skin exposed. When the figure is nominally female, it is made exceptionally active, even aggressive; when male, more passive, even sneaky; the females are given short hair, distinctive features; the males long hair and soft, hazy features – all merging towards (though not duplicating exactly) an androgynous oneness, the perfect erotic child.
>
> (Kincaid, 1992: 364)

Whether one fully accepts Kincaid's description or not, what he points to, as does the androgynous child of the mid-nineteenth century, is a tendency to see in the child an innocence and a purity that acquires its eroticism without recourse to gender. The otherness of the child lies not in gender but in its difference from adults and it is this difference which sexualises the child in the adult mind.

Gender and childhood: girls

If perceptions of masculinity were less clear-cut than is sometimes suggested, it is perhaps not surprising that perceptions of femininity should also suggest underlying uncertainties. The image of the feminine is made up of contradictions; the Victorian woman is economically dependent but morally strong; weak, but the maintainer of standards; rationally inferior but with greater intuitive sensitivity; sexually passive but (when awakened) sexually dangerous; aesthetically of less character but greater beauty. These contradictions, that were used to define the private, domestic sphere as woman's only proper realm, and at the same time to give it depth and power, frequently found expression in Victorian poetry. The following is from an anonymous, probably female poet's verse entitled 'Women's Rights', which first appeared in the magazine *Temple Bar*:

> A Woman's rights. What do these words convey?
> What depths of old-world wisdom do they reach?

What is their real intent? O sister say;
And strive in daily life their truth to teach.

The right in others' joys a joy to find;
A right divine to weep when others weep;
The right to be all unceasing kind:
The right to wake and pray while others sleep.

To be little children's truest friend,
To know them in their ever-changing mood;
Forgetting self to labour to the end
To be a gracious influence for good.

The right in strength and honours to be free;
In daily work accomplished finding rest!
The right in 'trivial round' a sphere to see;
The right in blessing to be fully blest.
(Cole and Hope, n.d.)

Such high flown sentiments were probably for an adult audience – or perhaps for that time when female adolescent sensibilities were thought ripe for such encounters with destiny. As Gorham has shown, there is often a harder edge to the upbringing of girls than these sentiments would suggest. In economic conditions which were never entirely secure for much of the middle classes, girls needed emotional skills of a high order as well as practical common sense (Gorham, 1982; see also Burstyn, 1980; Dyhouse, 1981). Another anonymous poem deals not with women's rights but with 'Girls That Are In Demand', and the tone whilst bearing some of the same rhetoric as the previous poem has also a more down to earth ring about it, as befits its underlying economic assumptions:

The girls that are wanted are good girls –
Good from the heart to the lips;
Pure as the lily is white and pure,
From its heart to its sweet leaf tips.
The girls that are wanted are home girls –
Girls that are mother's right hand
That fathers and brothers can trust to,
And the little ones understand.

Girls that are fair on the hearthstone,

And pleasant when nobody sees;
Kind and sweet to their own folks
Ready and anxious to please.
The girls that are wanted are wise girls,
That know what to do and to say;
That drive with a smile and a soft word
The wrath of the household away.

The girls that are wanted are girls of sense,
Whom fashions can never deceive;
Who can follow whatever is pretty,
And dare what is silly to leave.
The girls that are wanted are careful girls,
Who count what a thing will cost,
Who use with a prudent generous hand,
But see that nothing is lost.

The girls that are wanted are girls with hearts;
They are wanted for mothers and wives,
Wanted to cradle in loving arms
The strongest and frailest lives.
The clever, the witty, the brilliant girl,
There are few who can understand;
But, Oh! for the wise, loving home girls
There's a steady constant demand.

(Cole and Hope, n.d.)

What gives coherence to the contradictions is that most of them are captured and held by the notion of femininity, a concept that Gorham argues began with the Enlightenment (not least with Rousseau's Sophie) and found its full flowering in the Victorian age. But it was with female sexuality that the concept of the feminine found its greatest difficulty. As Gorham says, 'The ideal of feminine purity is implicitly asexual; how, then, could it be reconciled with the active sexuality that would inevitably be included in the duties of wife and mother?' (Gorham, 1982: 7).

One solution to this problem suggested by Gorham is that the ideal of the feminine was focused particularly upon the daughter rather than the wife or mother, and upon the child rather than the adult. Upon the image of the girl, especially in relation to her father and her brothers, could be projected purity, dependence, and a sense of duty and devotion. And there was no need for adult sexuality to cast its shadow over the 'sunbeam' of the family (ibid.: 7, 38). There is no better portrait of these sunbeams than in the stories of Daisy Ashford, born in 1881, whose literary career lasted from approximately 1885 to 1895. This child author, best known for the exploits of Ethel and Mr Salteena in *The Young Visiters*, wrote a number of stories in which childish preoccupations are infused with an anticipation of adult life and, in particular, with the excitements of romance and marriage and the duties that lie the other side of marriage. There is an example, too, in 'The Hangman's Daughter', of an adoring daughter and of a brother as rescuing hero. Indeed her collected works provide a fascinating glimpse of the way in which Victorian discourses about the feminine were absorbed by one precocious middle-class child (Ashford, 1919, 1983). They show, too, some of its many contradictions; the strictures relating to manners and to morality (Daisy's upbringing was Roman Catholic), the fantasies of romantic love that dominate several of the stories and the staggering ease with which romantic love is allowed to glide into the responsibilities of motherhood. In Chapter 9 of *The Young Visiters*, for example, Bernard the hero of the story takes Ethel boating. He rows whilst she 'lay among the rich cushions of the dainty boat', but Ashford adds rather tartly, 'She had rather a lazy nature but Bernard did not know of this'. In due course Bernard proposes:

> Oh Bernard muttered Ethel this is so sudden.
>
> No no cried Bernard and taking the bull by both horns he kissed her violently on her dainty face. My bride to be he murmured several times.
>
> Ethel trembled with joy as she heard these mistick words . . .
>
> (Ashford, 1919)

After a Marriage at Westminster Abbey (Ethel wrote out the invitations herself) the happy couple go on honeymoon to Egypt for six weeks, from whence they return 'with a son and hair a nice fat baby called Ignatius Bernard'. With unfailing generosity, the author grants the new parents, 'six more children four boys and three girls and some of them were twins which was very exciting'.

The happy domestic scene, to which the daughters had such a vital contribution to make and which inspired many paintings especially from early Victorian artists, had, as Roberts remarks, a reality behind it; the close family life providing the framework for a happy, if clearly defined and strictly policed, childhood (Roberts, 1972). However, as

Manheimer graphically puts it, 'the Angel in the House was caught in a dialectical dance with the demons at the door', and from the darkness outside came images which disturbed the sense of seamless continuity between girl and adult that Daisy Ashford so effortlessly assumed (Manheimer, 1979).

Outside the bourgeois home, increasingly suburban with its secluded gardens, lay the 'nether regions' some distance away in the sprawling urban jungles of the rapidly growing cities. Davidoff has shown how the organic conception of society which gained currency in the second half of the nineteenth century viewed middle-class man as the head, his wife as the heart and the soul, and the industrial manual workers as the hands who were the 'unthinking, unfeeling "doers", without characteristics of sex, age, or other identity' (Davidoff, 1979: 89). Following such bodily metaphors the poor, the criminals, the destitute of the cities were the offal, the effluvia, a threat to the sanitary bourgeois world. Into this category came prostitutes who threatened the physical and the moral health of the middle classes. Some saw prostitution as 'a necessary institution which acted as a giant sewer, drawing away the distasteful but inevitable waste products of male lustfulness, leaving the middle-class household and middle-class ladies pure and unsullied' (ibid.: 89). But the separation could never be absolute; the bourgeois woman was a sexual being and the prostitute was still a woman, the Madonna and the Magdalene shared the same basic human nature.

Not even the female child could escape this duality and there was a voyeurism amongst the Victorians, in respect of both the Madonna and the Magdalene, that disturbed the settled image of domesticated femininity. According to Nina Auerbach,

> While right-thinking Victorians were elevating woman into an angel, their art slithered with images of a mermaid. Angels were thought to be meekly self-sacrificial by nature: in this cautiously diluted form, they were pious emblems of a good woman's submergence in her family. Mermaids, on the other hand, submerge themselves not to negate their power but to conceal it.
>
> (Auerbach, 1982: 7)

Whilst the image of the angel was feminised and sentimentalised to capture and control it (biblical angels, after all, are male), the power of the mermaid, always essentially feminine, escaped domestic control and threatened the social order. Hans Christian Andersen wrote *The Little Mermaid* in the 1830s, and from the 1840s this and his other stories began to appear in English translations. *The Little Mermaid* tells of the youngest of six daughters of the Sea King emerging from childhood to adult sexual awareness and thence through death to angelic immortality. As a child she falls in love with the image of boy, a statue fallen from a wrecked ship to the bottom of the sea. When each child reaches the age of 15, they emerge from their childhoods and are allowed to rise to the surface to gaze upon the world of men, a world described by Andersen as richly sensuous and exotic.

When eventually her turn comes, the youngest child is dressed by her grandmother with the ornaments of her adult sexual status, constraints which hurt but which must be borne. Rising to the surface she finds a great ship and on it a Prince with whom she falls in love. The ship is wrecked, but she saves the Prince and takes him safely to the shore without his knowledge. There he is found by a girl from a nearby convent. Unable to forget him, the Little Mermaid visits the sea witch and in exchange for her tongue she is given a magic draught that will cut her fishes tail in two, as if she were cut with a sharp sword. Now voiceless, but a sexually complete human being, she is discovered naked by the Prince at the entrance to his palace. The sea witch has told her that if she can make him love her, she will gain an immortal soul; if she fails, at the moment he marries another, her heart will break and she will become foam upon the surface of the sea. With all the sensuality at her command, she woos him, dancing for him although her feet feel as though they are cut with knives at every step. The Prince loves her, kisses her lips and plays with her long hair, but loves her as a child, not as a wife. Himself in love with the girl from the convent, he discovers that she is the Princess his parents want him to marry. Facing death the Little Mermaid is offered a knife by her sisters and with it the chance to save herself by killing the Prince, but she throws the knife away and is dissolved into sea foam. However, she rises from the foam to become a daughter of the air. Her sensuality is replaced by an ethereal spirituality and she is offered the chance to gain an immortal soul by a 100 years of good works. But the success of this task is dependent upon the behaviour of children; a good child reduces the time by a year, but a bad child brings tears to the daughters of air and each tear adds a day to the 100 years.

Andersen's fable is a far cry from the smooth transition from girlhood to womanhood recited so faithfully by the young Daisy Ashford. And yet this tale, with its desperate yearnings, its rich sensuality and its earthly tragedy (which so outweighs its ethereal and very bourgeois conclusion) was perhaps also part of Daisy's childhood experience, and it captures a mythology of Victorian female sexuality not easily dismissed. As Auerbach, again says,

> Andersen's mermaid clings winsomely to her dispossession, but her choice is a guide to a vital Victorian mythology whose lovable woman is a silent and self-disinherited mutilate, the fullness of whose extraordinary and dangerous being might at any moment return through violence. The taboos that encased the Victorian woman contained buried tributes to her disruptive power.
>
> (Auerbach, 1982: 8)

Through Andersen's own voyeurism, the little girl who read the story of the Little Mermaid might sense a gaze which viewed her own incipient sexuality as an imperative, dominating, dangerous force to be curbed, confined and held within the realm of childhood.

CHILD PROSTITUTION AND THE CASE OF ELIZA ARMSTRONG

There was no unified perception of prostitution amongst the Victorians. On the one hand there were those like William Acton (his book, *Prostitution*, was first published in 1857) who took a broadly economic rationalist view of prostitution. This view presented the prostitute as a hard-headed entrepreneur, calculating upon the limited opportunities of her situation, who enjoyed the gay life she led and who, in all probability, would eventually settle down and marry as successfully as most (Mason, 1994b: 85; Walkowitz, 1980: 42). The journalist Henry Mayhew found one such, who scorned his question as to what would become of her, with the sharp response: 'What an absurd question. I could marry tomorrow if I liked' (quoted Auerbach, 1982: 159). Mayhew's colleague Bracebridge Hemyng also found a category of 'the happy prostitute . . . the thoroughly hardened, clever infidel . . . who in the end seldom fails to marry well' (quoted Mason, 1994b: 85). On the other hand, there were the Magdalenists, who saw the prostitute as victim, seduced by male lust and her own weakness, in need of rescue and moral and spiritual rehabilitation. Religiously inspired, and particularly the province of evangelical and dissenting circles, the Magdalenists took to the streets to rescue the prostitute, and having rescued her, they offered asylum but demanded penitence. Cutting across these perceptions, especially towards the end of the century, were feminist reformers like Josephine Butler who combined a deep sense of sin with a strong sense of the rights of adult women to determine their own lives, and who linked anti-sensualism with a rational feminism.

In the last third of the century, several factors brought debates about prostitution to a head. An attempt to regulate prostitution and control venereal disease, through the enforced examination of women suspected of prostitution, was made through the Contagious Diseases Acts, the first of which became law in 1864 (Walkowitz, 1980). Associated with the military (they applied only to towns with a strong military presence) and also with privilege and loose morality, the Acts were increasingly opposed by various groups with a radical and sometimes evangelical orientation, not least by the Ladies National Association for the Repeal of the Contagious Diseases Acts, founded in 1869. It was in this organisation that Josephine Butler's charismatic personality found its public voice. Her sympathetic identification with the working-class women who were the objects of the Acts, her description of the medical inspection as 'instrumental rape', and her rage against the double standard of sexual morality which the Acts implicitly condoned raised the emotional temperature of the debates considerably.

From the midst of these debates grew the Social Purity organisations, some of which were to last beyond the end of the Second World War, and which, perhaps more than anything else, carried the concept of Victorian sexual prudery to the twentieth-century imagination. The environmentalism which had such an influence over social reform in mid-century began to give way again to a revived evangelicism which emphasised depravity rather than deprivation (Weeks, 1981: 81f; Mason, 1994a: 251). Mason is quite clear about the overall impact of the Social Purity movements of the late nineteenth century:

> The Social Purity Alliance was a grotesque affair, a great bubble of extreme anti-sensualism whose only lasting achievement was to discredit sexual moralism. In fact, it is surely this episode of last-gasp, hypertrophied asceticism, occurring at the very end of Victoria's reign, which very largely explains the very swift establishment of the 'Victorian' as a stigmatizing label in the first twenty years of the next century.
>
> (Mason, 1994b: 213)

One of the issues which gave impetus to the Social Purity movement was child prostitution. In mid-century, as Kincaid has noted, even though many prostitutes were probably young, the child as prostitute was not central to the debate (Kincaid, 1992: 77). In the last third of the century this began to change. Child prostitution gained currency as a public issue in the context of the opposition to the Contagious Diseases Acts. Because of the generally heightened consciousness about prostitution and about the morality which allowed prostitution to flourish, a moral panic about child prostitution was almost inevitable. As in most states of moral panic, facts are hard to come by. Some recent scholars, like Walkowitz, believe the extent of child prostitution was probably exaggerated, though Smith has cautioned against too much scepticism (Walkowitz, 1980; Smith, 1979: 303). In mid-century, Acton had taken his usual line, noting the 'extreme youth of the junior portion of the "street-walkers"', but was unconvinced by the view that they were victims of a depraved upper class. Loss of virginity occurred mostly with boys of their own age and class and was a 'natural consequence of promiscuous herding' amongst the lower classes (quoted Kincaid, 1992: 77). But as moral, evangelical views gained in influence, child prostitution moved centre stage and, amidst stories of young girls being sold for prostitution at home, or shipped off to continental brothels, agitation began for legislation to raise the age of consent. The intention was to criminalise the procuring and use of girls for prostitution. In fact, in 1861 the age of consent was raised from 10 to 12, in 1875 it was raised to 13 and in 1885, the year when the issue reached its most sensational stage, it was raised to 16. The importance of this whole episode lies not simply in the social and moral reforms which were at issue, but also in the way in which definitions of childhood became closely related to sexuality. The age of consent became an important symbolic definition of the end of childhood, especially in relation to girls; the moment when the innocence of childhood ended and entry into the world of the adult began. It was, however, a definition which took no account of the social and economic circumstances of the girls in question.

The issue came to a head with the intervention of the journalist and editor of the campaigning *Pall Mall Gazette*, W.T. Stead. Legislation to raise the age of consent was before parliament but had stalled in the face of opposition. Through his connections with several people campaigning against child prostitution, including Benjamin Waugh, the founder of the National Society for the Prevention of Cruelty to Children, and Josephine Butler herself, Stead was drawn into the campaign. In what is now one of the most famous and infamous pieces of Victorian investigative journalism, Stead set out to prove his case by actually demonstrating that it was possible, in London, to purchase a young girl for the purpose of prostitution. With the aid of

Josephine Butler and of Bramwell Booth of the Salvation Army, the girl he bought was the 13-year-old Eliza Armstrong. At Stead's behest she was purchased by Rebecca Jarrett, a former prostitute known to Josephine Butler, and taken to a midwife-cum-abortionist who examined her and testified to her virginity. Then she was taken to a room in a brothel and given chloroform. Shortly afterwards Stead entered, but Eliza was still awake and cried out, whereupon Stead immediately left the room. The next day Bramwell Booth arranged for her to be taken to France and a position found for her there. This story was the centre-piece of a series of articles in the *Pall Mall Gazette* which went under the banner of 'The Maiden Tribute of Modern Babylon'.

Through the intense publicity that these revelations generated, through press rivalry which sought to discredit their author and through an element of sheer chance, Stead was subsequently brought to trial and convicted of abduction and of aiding and abetting indecent assault. He was jailed, an event he gloried in, wearing his prison clothes on every anniversary of his incarceration. In the midst of the controversy that raged around the publication of Stead's revelations, parliament, in the Criminal Law Amendment Act of 1885, raised the age of consent to 16. The details of this extraordinary episode, the buying of the child, the press campaign in the *Pall Mall Gazette*, and the aftermath of Stead's trial and imprisonment are well told elsewhere (Barry, 1979; Petrie, 1971; Plowden, 1974; Schultz, 1972). It is a story that has much to tell about the Victorian press, about late nineteenth-century parliamentary politics and the class conflicts embedded therein; about the nature of campaigning social reform and about the effectiveness of one committed, if arrogant, individual. But it also says much about the perceptions of childhood which were implicit in the whole episode.

This feature of the debate has been discussed most illuminatingly by Deborah Gorham, who sees in the campaign against child prostitution not much evidence of clear-sighted purpose and a great deal of confused and muddled perceptions (Gorham, 1978). The confusion arose particularly in relation to childhood sexuality. Given that one of the main driving forces behind the campaign was bourgeois evangelical religious enthusiasm, it is inevitable that there was an emphasis upon personal morality as opposed to environmental circumstances. Couple this with the fact that reformers brought with them to the campaign a bourgeois conception of domesticity, femininity and childhood, with its associated perceptions of female sexual passivity, and it is not surprising, as Gorham says, that the 'reformers were not fully able to confront the way in which sexuality was conditioned by age, sex and social class' (ibid.: 356). Ignoring the realities of working-class life and working with an ideal image of the young girl depicted in poems like 'Girls That Are In Demand', they could hardly fail to see the child prostitute as the victim of degenerate, aristocratic male lust. In this the Social Purity campaigners found common ground not only with radicals like Stead, but also with feminist anti-sensualists like Josephine Butler.

The law on the age of consent was seen as a measure to protect the defenceless, but as Gorham points out, many working-class girls who casually engaged in illicit sex or even prostitution did not see it that way. In any case, she argues, from a bourgeois perspective, protection had much to do with controlling the sexuality of the growing child (ibid.: 364). It is worth noting that some of the Social Purity campaigners wanted the age of consent to be raised to 18 or even 21. Even Josephine Butler, who so vigorously opposed the Contagious Diseases Acts on the grounds that they infringed upon the liberty of working-class women, could not deny the call to protect the helpless child. Indeed, one of the overwhelming impressions left by the whole debate is that the symbol of the child was being used, not simply to legislate in the child's own defence, but also to assert the right of a moral majority to regulate the behaviour of all children in the interests of a particular ideology. It was, as several more recent commentators have pointed out, an episode driven less by moral reformers with a radical edge and more by groups who saw in child prostitution a sign of general moral decline (Walkowitz, 1980; Weeks, 1981; Mason, 1994b). At the centre of the campaign was a muddled image which has become so characteristic of late twentieth-century anxieties, the precocious child who is both victim of and threat to society.

What gave the moral majority its force in this argument, and enabled it to incorporate people like Stead and Butler, was the power of the late Victorian symbolism of the female. Perhaps because, as Gorham argues, the Victorians did not have a fully developed psycho-social definition of adolescence, they found it difficult to conceptualise the problem of teenage sexuality in the way which has become customary in the twentieth century (Gorham, 1978: 369). Rather they dealt in images that were black and white. On the one hand was the child of innocence, the ideal daughter of the bourgeois household, dependent upon parents, sexually unaware perhaps, but in terms of gender acutely conscious of the different emotional and social roles allotted to men and women. On the other hand, there was the precocious girl epitomised by the child prostitute whose innocence had been destroyed by her engagement in the sexual act. In such a creature all the darker forces of female sexuality were gathered; she was dangerous, out of control, and above all a threat to the status and honour that should properly be accorded to the angel in the house. It was the definition of the young prostitute as child which was the uniting issue. In the past, the Magdalenists had occasionally been able to find a common sisterhood between the bourgeois reformer and the adult prostitute, and late nineteenth- and early twentieth-century feminism could attempt to unite women around an anti-sensualist agenda that, in Christabel Pankhurst's slogan, demanded not only votes for women but also chastity for men (Walkowitz, 1980, 1982; Jeffreys, 1985). But to admit the female child to such a sisterhood was beyond the imagination even of a Josephine Butler. Sympathetic acknowledgement of the realities of life and of prostitution as a rational response to it had no place in discussions of the female child whatever her circumstances. The precocious working-class child was to be denied legitimate sexuality, and even though termed a helpless victim, she was to be incarcerated in reformatory or industrial school, where every move, every utterance, every gesture would be monitored and checked in an attempt, usually fruitless, to return her to her childhood (Gorham, 1978: 373). The experience of the bourgeois child was, no doubt, in many ways much happier; privilege and protection were not to be despised. But the principle role of the young Victorian bourgeois child was to nurture in her own person the contradictory powers of the angel and of the fallen woman, to absorb the morality and the sensuality of a tale like Andersen's *The Little Mermaid* and to offer to the world a potent innocence in which the denial of sexuality, in true Foucauldian manner, served not to repress but rather to enhance its power.

THE CULT OF THE LITTLE GIRL

'Innocence', remarks Kincaid, 'is not . . . detected but granted, not nurtured but enforced; it comes at the child as a denial of a whole host of capacities, an emptying out' (Kincaid, 1992: 73). And having been, as Kincaid puts it, 'emptied out', the child can be filled with whatever qualities adults choose to favour. Into the little girl were poured qualities of innocence which, though they could be shared by boys to some degree, acquired a special potency in the little girl through the power of her incipient sexuality. In what is frequently termed 'the cult of the little girl', these qualities were reverenced and expressed in terms which to the late twentieth-century mind are often disturbing. Three men frequently crop up in discussions of this cult and we shall use them as a focus for this brief discussion; they are Francis Kilvert, John Ruskin and Lewis Carroll.

Francis Kilvert was a clergyman who, during the 1870s, wrote a detailed and extensive diary of his daily life, thoughts and imaginings. What is characteristic of Kilvert and of the others in this discussion is their adoration of the naked or partially unclothed child. Nor apparently were parents always reluctant to show off their offspring. One mother, Kilvert recalled, undressed her little boy for his benefit 'so as to shew his bottom and thighs naked from the waist downward'. Sometimes the child was willing, but adults intervened. Polly, about to get in the bath tub, undressed to her drawers, apparently at Kilvert's request, and would have taken these off too had her grandmother not prevented her. Not that it made much difference since the article of clothing in question was clearly inadequate and Kilvert was able to enjoy 'a most interesting view from the rear'. Sometimes it was mere accident that granted Kilvert his view of forbidden flesh. A little girl at a fair got her clothes caught on the seat of a swing and it became apparent to the onlookers that she had no drawers on at all. Her modesty was discreetly re-established, but Kilvert was left with a happy memory of flesh that was 'plump and smooth and in excellent whipping condition'.

In these incidents from everyday life, it is the sensuousness of the flesh that attracts Kilvert. In his imaginings, however, it is more a conventional female beauty that captures him and his descriptions, as Kincaid notes, slip from the 'erotic to the soapy-pious':

> How is the indescribable beauty of that most lovely face to be described – the dark soft curls parting back from the pure white transparent brow, the exquisite little mouth and pearly tiny teeth, the long dark fringes and white eyelids that droop over and curtain her eyes . . . and seem to rest upon the soft clear cheek, and when the eyes are raised, that clear unfathomable blue depth of wide wonder and enquiry and unsullied and unsuspecting innocence. Oh, child, child if you did but know your own power. Oh, Gipsy, if you grow up as good as you are fair. Oh, that you might grow up good. May all God's angels guard you, sweet. The Lord bless thee and keep thee. The Lord make his face to shine upon thee and be gracious

> unto thee. The Lord lift up his countenance upon thee . . . both now and evermore. Amen.
>
> (quotations from Kincaid, 1992: 240ff; Pearsall, 1983: 445)

There is a striking, almost incongruous contrast between this very conventional, if plainly erotic writing that merges into the incantations of the preacher and the frank enjoyment of bare flesh, especially buttocks, in the cottage kitchen or village fair. But to Kilvert they seem to merge one into the other in an unequivocal adoration of the all that is beautiful and sensuous in childhood. What is hidden from us, because Kilvert will not tell us, is the meaning with which all this is imbued. It is an iconography of childhood which still has meaning in the late twentieth century in a certain jokiness about young children's immodest nakedness and in the now heavily commercialised veneration of young, childlike female beauty. But the emotion is distrusted, and has been consigned to the realm of the paedophile. Hence, as Kincaid notes, we are at something of a loss to understand:

> How much awareness Kilvert allowed himself of the nature of interests like these we cannot know, just as we cannot be sure what exactly his consciousness of such matters really could amount to. He does not generally reflect upon these points; we could not hear him very well had he done so. What is clear is that he did not regard these children lightly.
>
> (Kincaid, 1992: 242)

John Ruskin made plain his very orthodox, bourgeois perception of the feminine in his description of the role of women in his essay 'Of Queen's Gardens'. This was first delivered as a lecture in 1864 and according to Kate Millett offers 'one of the most complete insights obtainable into that compulsive masculine fantasy one might call the official Victorian attitude' (Millett, 1972: 122). Women, because of their natures, claims Ruskin, should occupy a separate sphere of activity and influence, and adopt an attitude of self-renunciation in their service to family and society. Their education should be more concerned with sentiment than with reason and, like Wordsworth's child of nature, they should grow naturally and blossom like the flower. It is against this perception of women in general that Ruskin's view of little girls should be seen. Leaving aside his own infatuations, the clearest evidence of his ideal is to be found in his attitude to the work of the artist Kate Greenaway. She specialised in drawings of children in rural English landscapes, especially little girls who mostly look as if they have strayed into the late nineteenth century from the end of the eighteenth. To say, as not infrequently it is suggested, that they have escaped from a Jane Austen novel is a calumny against Austen's own very realistic and sober accounts of childhood, but clearly, even in Greenaway's own times, they were deliberate anachronisms (Pearsall, 1983; Holme, 1976). Amongst the poems for which Greenaway provided illustrations were those of the Taylor sisters, whose poetry had been an important part of her own childhood reading. Ruskin was sufficiently captured by the style of illustration employed by Greenaway and similar artists and illustrators like Mrs Allingham that he devoted one of his lectures (during his second tenure of the Oxford University Slade Professorship) largely to the work of these two. After noting the absence of children from Greek and from Gothic art Ruskin claims,

> But from the moment when the spirit of Christianity has been entirely interpreted to the Western races, the sanctity of womanhood worshipped in the Madonna, and the sanctity of childhood in unity with that of Christ, became the light of every honest hearth, and the joy of every pure and chastened soul.
>
> (quoted Salway, 1976: 239)

Thus a tradition of literary and pictorial representation of children developed, was briefly buried by the insidious effects of the industrial revolution, but then re-emerged through Wordsworth and Dickens,

> till at last, bursting out like one of the sweet Surrey fountains, all dazzling and pure, you have the radiance and innocence of reinstated infant divinity showered again among the flowers of English meadows by Mrs Allingham and Kate Greenaway.
>
> (ibid.: 240)

But, as with Kilvert, there is more to Ruskin's admiration than this uncritical, fulsome praise for an artist who touched (and still does a hundred years later) a strand of intense sentimentality about children. In a letter to Greenaway, Ruskin commented about one drawing, 'As we've got as far as taking off hats, I trust we may in time get to taking off just a little more – say, mittens – and then – perhaps – even shoes! – and (for fairies) even stockings – and then –' (quoted Holme, 1976: 10). This goes beyond mere sentimentality and, as with Kilvert, suggests a desire for the erotic gaze to be turned upon the child. The difference is that Kilvert felt no need to pretend that the erotic was to be found in the land of fairies.

Lewis Carroll, perhaps the most famous figure in relationship to the cult of the little girl, presents initially a similar picture to Ruskin. Pearsall recounts how Carroll bombarded Harry Furniss, the illustrator of *Sylvie and Bruno*, with suggestions about models for the illustrations and about how they should be dressed:

> I *wish* I dared dispense with all costume; naked children are so perfectly pure and lovely, but . . . it would never do. . . . Bare legs and feet we *must* have, at any rate. . . . As to your Sylvie. I am charmed with your idea of dressing her in *white*; it exactly fits my own idea of her; I want her to be a sort of embodiment of Purity.
>
> (quoted Pearsall, 1983: 431)

Carroll, in correspondence with Furniss, also referred to his friend, Miss E. Gertrude Thomson who illustrated his *Three Sunsets and Other Poems* as being an 'artist great in fairies'. According to Pearsall, Miss Thomson was once called to book even by Christina Rossetti for the indecency of her fairies, but her drawings would seem to represent Carroll's ideal, long-haired, angelic features, butterfly wings and, of course, completely unclothed and very evidently composed in such a way as to display their nakedness to best advantage. With Carroll there is once again this mixture of the sentimental, the fey and the religious, together with a sensuousness which is inescapably erotic. Inevitably with Carroll, however, it is never quite so simple because the gaze is often returned by the little girls themselves. Sylvie is an invention of an imagination long past its prime and she certainly is a passive creature. According to Briggs and Butts, she is less a descendant of Alice than a 'dream-child and object of unacknowledged desire' whose legacy is with Barrie's *Peter Pan* (Briggs and Butts, 1995: 141).

But before Sylvie came the far more forceful Alice, both the Alice of the stories and the real Alice Liddell of the photographs. The Alice of the two books, *Alice in Wonderland* and *Alice Through the Looking Glass*, is such a powerful and rich symbol that she has, particularly in recent years, been the subject of the kind of intense scrutiny normally reserved for adult fiction (Empson, 1935; Phillips, 1972; Kincaid, 1973; Guiliano, 1982; Carpenter, 1985; Auerbach, 1982, 1986; Batchelor, 1989; Grey, 1992). In terms of how we should view Alice, opinion is divided. At one end of the spectrum is Batchelor who denies that questions of adolescence and female sexuality have anything to do with the Alice stories:

> She is *not* adolescent. The Alice books are about learning, not about sexual growth: the person engaged in power-struggles in the two books, and who grows intellectually and socially – very fast – remains a seven year old girl.
>
> (Batchelor, 1989: 182)

Such a view has its merits, especially if the stories are read (as twentieth-century readers are quite entitled to read them) without reference to their Victorian context. Nor is it really a matter of Carroll's intent and motivation since he, no more than Kilvert or even Ruskin, could never interpret his own response to little girls in a way that would satisfy a twentieth-century listener. It is less a question of interpretation than of seeing what resonances Carroll's Alice has with other Victorian discourses about femininity. In this respect, Nina Auerbach again has something of interest to say. In her discussion of the development of the myth of the fallen woman, Auerbach identifies Alice with the fallen, not to deny her innocence, but to suggest how inextricably interwoven were the dual images of woman as angel and woman as whore. Auerbach suggests that when the spirituality of the angel entered the fallen woman, she acquired a potency, a perversity which disturbed, but which was also part of what Kate Millett called that 'compulsive male fantasy'. Little girls could also be caught up in this duality, and hence for Auerbach the Alice books are inevitably concerned with womanhood:

> Carroll's book may seem a surprising addition to our adult context, but in so potent a cultural myth, one containing so many intense and unexamined feelings about womanhood, it should not surprise us if extremes meet, and the demonic energy of the fallen woman shares some of the preternatural purity Carroll located in little girls.
>
> (Auerbach, 1982: 167)

Elsewhere Auerbach suggests that it is through a (no doubt unconscious) perception of the myth of fallen womanhood that Carroll enables Alice to escape from the soporific normality of her everyday existence:

> Like Milton's Eve, the ever-ravenous Alice is a creature of curiosity and appetite. Eve fell through eating to become a god, and Alice, who is always hungry, becomes the creator of worlds through falling. As her curiosity causes her fall, so her hunger impels her rise: eating and drinking produce the size changes that at times

> place her at the mercy of Wonderland but ultimately allow her to rule it. In this loving parody of Genesis and of contemporary fallen women, Alice is simultaneously Wonderland's slave and its queen, its creator and destroyer as well as its victim. Carroll's pure little girl, so painfully aware of her etiquette, takes much of her paradoxical power from an army of women whose activities she would not have been allowed to know.... Carroll's peculiarly Victorian triumph lay in his amalgamation of the fallen woman with the unfallen child.
>
> (Auerbach, 1986: 152)

And what of the photographs, especially those few of nude girls? Cohen is right to assert the futility of trying to read from them what sexual fantasies Carroll had about little girls (Cohen, 1984: 3). There is no doubt, however, that Carroll was conscious of the possible misconstruction that could be put upon his friendships for young girls. His sister Mary once questioned the propriety of these relationships, and Carroll replied:

> The only two tests I now apply to such a question as the having some particular girl-friend as a guest are, first, my own *conscience*, to settle whether I feel it to be entirely innocent and right in the sight of God; secondly, the *parents* of my friend, to settle whether I have their *full* approval for what I do.... If you limit your actions in life to things that *nobody* can possibly find fault with, you will not do much!
>
> (quoted Cohen, 1984: 14)

He was also, as Cohen shows, very articulate in his defence of his wish to photograph some of his subjects 'without any drapery or suggestion of it'. He asserted his 'deep sense of admiration for *form*, especially the human form' as 'the most beautiful thing God has made on this earth'. The photographs, he asserted to the parents of a potential model, should be 'such as you might if you liked frame and hang up in your drawing-room'. He would not ask, he said, 'if I thought there was any fear of its lessening *their* [the child's] simplicity of character' (quoted ibid.: 15). However, whilst Cohen is right to challenge a late twentieth-century prurience, that cannot be entirely the end of the story. 'Innocence', 'simplicity', 'purity', all words Carroll uses in relation to girls, are words that can, as Auerbach suggests and Carroll's own Alice so animatedly demonstrates, mask a potency quite at odds with the passivity so often associated with them.

Later in life, they lost that power for Carroll, but at the time of the Alice stories and of the photographs (mostly from the 1860s and 1870s) childhood innocence did represent something of power and energy.

Carol Mavor has argued that there is no point in trying to 'veil the obvious sexuality that Carroll captured on the photographic plates' or in trying to wash out the contradictions inherent in his treatment of the female child (Mavor, 1994: 157). Cohen tends to see Carroll as repressed, and attributes his repression to his Victorian orthodoxy, but whilst such an explanation gets us beyond individualistic interpretations, it relies perhaps too heavily upon the twentieth-century myth of the upright Victorian male. If we follow Auerbach, of course, the contradiction lies not in the individual personality of Carroll, but in the broader cultural perception of the Victorian woman with its duality of Madonna and Magdalene. Mavor takes this as a starting point but points to an added complication when the female in question is a young child.

The period when Carroll was taking his photographs was the period running up to the campaigns about child prostitution we have already discussed. Implicit in those campaigns was a wish to categorise the female child as sexless, to divide the innocent female child from even the possibility of sexual knowledge. It is perhaps this desire that Carroll reflected when he insisted on preserving the 'simplicity' of the child's character. But, Mavor argues, in the photographed child (such as in the famous nude photograph of the 7-year-old Evelyn Hatch) the child represents for Carroll a creature whose difference is marked, not merely in terms of gender, but also in her very possession of the state of childhood. And in that state of childhood, she becomes again the primitive, the child of nature, not Millais' or Greenaway's nostalgic mob-capped icons of a lost rural Eden, but 'neological: sexual and sexualized, childlike and womanly, innocent and knowing' (Mavor, 1994: 165). Once more we seem to be in the world of Romanticism, of Fairchild's 'sublime confusion of the physical and the metaphysical' in which the power of Nature itself is manifest in the child (Fairchild, 1961: 378). In this sense Evelyn Hatch is heir, not so much to a repressed and prurient Victorianism, but rather to Wordsworth's Lucy who was granted so short a life, and before Lucy to Andrew Marvell's little *T.C.*, that 'virtuous Enemy of Man' who must be appeased, but whose potency was so fragile and delicate. In Carroll 's photographs, as in his writings, Carroll sought to capture the moment of childhood, but it was a moment, as Mavor has shown, full of contradictions for him. What is most remarkable about the Carroll of the period of the Alice books is the way in which his fictive Alice can view the world with such clarity and honesty. Similarly the little girls in his photographs gaze back at the photographer with such candour and lack of fear that the art within the photograph is as much their art as his (Mavor, 1994). But Carroll could not escape the determining cultural context of the cult of the little girl by which he was surrounded and, as he grew older, the saccharine images, so evident in *Sylvie and Bruno*, became dominant, and Mavor is undoubtedly right to see his photographic images as atypical for the age. Perhaps also she is right to see, in spite of the candour, a flicker of indecision in the faces of the little girls themselves, 'caught, with the Victorian girl, in an act of blushing and nonblushing at the same time'; the child, like Carroll himself, could not entirely escape Ruskin's 'official Victorian attitude'. What Carroll captured, as no other Victorian did, and captured because of his extraordinary empathy with and insight into the life of the Victorian little girl, was the sheer power and force of childhood innocence (ibid.: 188).

What perhaps, above all, the later Victorians granted to childhood was an aesthetic quality and a sensuousness that the twentieth century has never really come to terms with. In J.M. Barrie's novel *The Little White Bird*, the author-narrator describes the longed for day when his little friend David comes to stay the night with him. The chapter which describes this 'tremendous adventure' is filled with a nervous sensuality. The narrator pretends that putting a little boy to bed is an everyday occurrence to him, whilst in fact it is for him rather than for David that the experience is a real adventure.

> I placed him on my knee and removed his blouse. This was a delightful experience, but I think I remained wonderfully calm until I came somewhat too suddenly to his little braces, which agitated me profoundly.
>
> I cannot proceed in public with the disrobing of David.
>
> (Chapter 19)

In the night, David, lying in his own little bed beside the author, wakes up:

> 'I don't take up very much room,' the far-away voice said.
>
> 'Why, David,' said I, sitting up, 'do you want to come into my bed?'

> 'Mother said I wasn't to want it unless you wanted it first,' he squeaked.
>
> 'It is what I have been wanting all the time,' said I, and then without more ado the little white figure rose and flung itself at me. For the rest of the night he lay on me and across me, and sometimes his feet were at the bottom of the bed and sometimes on the pillow, but he always retained possession of my finger, and occasionally he woke me to say that he was sleeping with me.
>
> (Chapter 19)

The twentieth century has become increasingly embarrassed by such writing and, especially in relation to Barrie, has tended to hide behind a defensively critical stance which accuses the writing of an excess of sentimentality and the writer of an over-bearing possessiveness (Kincaid, 1992: 279ff). It is the play of a grown man with a young child that the twentieth century finds so difficult to tolerate, or rather the sensuality that such play naturally generates. And yet for all the attempts post-Victorian society has made to sublimate the adult desire to respond to the sensuality of the child, it will not go away. It is not, of course, that the Victorians were free of such attempts at sublimation, but in figures like Kilvert, Ruskin, Barrie and especially Lewis Carroll there were some who were unafraid to voice their response to the physical beauty of childhood. In exploring the ambiguities and the contradictions that shaped their expression, especially in relation to the female child, we should not forget how dramatically direct they could be and how, most particularly in the case of Carroll, the child found a voice which cut through the 'innumerable institutional devices and discursive strategies' which Foucault insists were increasingly surrounding them (Foucault, 1984: 30). As that cockiest of J.M. Barrie's boys, Peter Pan, himself put it,

> No one is going to catch me, lady!

Chapter 7

The child of crisis

The end of childhood?

> On Thursday morning, Michael's birthday, Artie hanged himself from the shower curtain rod in his bathroom. Luckily the rod broke and he fell into the tub, winding up with concussion and an assortment of cuts and bruises. . . . Both Michael and Erica blamed themselves. . . . We weren't in a mood to celebrate but I gave Michael his birthday present anyway. . . . In less than two hours Michael and Erica each polished off another three drinks and were acting really dumb, singing school songs and laughing hysterically. . . . Erica got sick first, in the parking lot. . . . A few miles down the highway Michael heaved all over Erica, but she was so out of it she didn't notice. . . . My mother and father were very generous about helping them, because the truth is, they looked and smelled disgusting. . . . We got Michael to bed in the den and Erica to bed in my room. Then I went to the bathroom, sat on the toilet, and cried.
>
> Judy Blume, *Forever*

There is a pervasive sense that the state of childhood is in crisis in the late twentieth century. It would be wrong to say that this feeling is total since there are areas of social and cultural life in which childhood is celebrated with a gusto that has rarely been found before. There is, for example, that energetic search for the authentic child, conducted most famously in the work of Peter and Iona Opie with their unique studies of children's rhymes and games (Opie I. and P., 1959, 1969, 1985; Opie, I. 1993). A similar celebration of childhood is to be found in much contemporary writing for children, especially in the poetry of writers like Michael Rosen or in that most glorious flowering of the late twentieth century, the children's picture book. This has come of age in the last twenty years or so, ironically when faced with the competition of television, producing masterpieces such as Maurice Sendak's *Where the Wild Things Are* and *In the Night Kitchen*, Anthony Browne's *Bear Goes to Town* or *Through the Magic Mirror*, John Scieszka and Lane Smith's *The True Story of the 3 Little Pigs! by A.*

Wolf or *The Stinky Cheese Man and other Fairly Stupid Tales*, Janet and Allan Ahlberg's *The Jolly Postman*, and John Burningham's *Come away from the water, Shirley* or *Grandpa*, to name but a few. In their wit and their exuberance and in their empathy with childhood's experiences and perceptions, the creators of the best contemporary picture books would seem to exemplify a society which understands the nature and the needs of childhood and which can respond with an unrestrained and uncondescending imagination. It reflects a society prepared to play with the child and to let the child, through the book, play with the adult world, and to do so with confidence, unafraid that either child or adult is adopting a false or demeaning role.

In the realm of science, too, childhood with its needs has established itself as a central preoccupation. For medicine and psychology, both having roots going back into the nineteenth century and beyond, the twentieth century has provided an institutional, bureaucratic and professional superstructure beyond the imagining of any Victorian. The study of education, too, has achieved industrial proportions in recognition of its importance to the economic and social welfare of advanced societies. Even in sociology, the state of childhood has recently shown signs of breaking free from the family and of becoming a field of study in its own right (Jenks, 1982; James and Prout, 1990; Qvortrup, 1994). The belief in knowledge and in its power to improve the condition of childhood would appear, at least on the surface, to be undiminished and the flow of information and advice from the expert to the lay-person grows ever broader as the era of the CD-ROM, offering information on every aspect of child-rearing from nappy rash to sex education, comes ever closer.

Perhaps it was within the sphere of social policy that, in Britain especially, the second half of the twentieth century seemed to promise most to childhood, or at least where that promise was most clearly and distinctly articulated through legislation. During the period of the 'golden age of welfare' spanning the thirty years or so following the Second World War, there was a sense that the welfare of the child was under control. Of course there were anxieties about delinquency and about enduring pockets of poverty, but childhood seemed to have survived the greatest threat to its existence – the coming of industrial society. This threat had been seen predominantly in terms of the environmental threat of industrialisation itself and its accompanying process of urbanisation, with all the attendant consequences for the dependent child. The battles over health and hygiene in the home, over the provision of universal education and over the protection of the child from the worst effects of urban poverty, seemed winnable if not already won. The survival was something to celebrate and to be proud of. At the end of the 1940s especially Britain and America had also survived two world wars, their social fabric apparently strengthened rather than diminished; childhood had become something to treasure, something to enjoy. Whatever remaining problems there were could be coped with through a benign combination of economic growth, a stable family, a caring community and state-backed professional organisations with the power of science at their fingertips.

With utter conviction, the historians of British social policy for children could write of,

> a growing understanding and appreciation of the necessary conditions for human life, health and happiness based on scientific knowledge denied to our forbears . . . a belief incomprehensible to earlier generations that children are citizens who have social rights independent of their parent's rights which the state has a duty to protect.
>
> (Pinchbeck and Hewitt, 1973: 637)

And of the 1948 Children Act, one of that cluster of post-war pieces of legislation that defined the welfare state in Britain, Jean Heywood, herself deeply involved in the implementation of the Act, could claim that through the Act,

> the community . . . defined and accepted again obligations which it bears towards its defenceless and ineffective members, helping the child . . . to grow to achieve a place of worth in an enabling society.
>
> (Heywood, 1965: 183)

What changed to make such expressions of belief and confidence sound naive and self-deluding to those living in the last decade of the century? Were these writers, in fact, naive environmentalists who failed to see that the problem lay, not in the conditions in which children were reared, but in the fallibility of those whose task it was to rear them? And had they allowed a romantic notion of childhood's innocence to blind them to the underlying truth of the doctrine of original sin – the truth that children come into the world so egocentric in their perception and so ill-equipped to learn the wisdom of their elders that, even in the most benign of conditions, growing up is a hazardous and contingent business? Such judgements are not profitable. It is all too easy to promote essentialist arguments against anybody who identifies a moment of historical importance, and there is no doubt that writers like Pinchbeck and Hewitt and Jean Heywood rightly sensed and properly conveyed the feeling of a period when confidence about the future of child welfare in its broadest sense was at its height.

Is the problem then that their extrapolation of historic trends in economic growth, in political and social stability, and in the power of scientific knowledge to alleviate distress was over-optimistic? To some degree the answer to this is clearly yes. Whilst it is possible to over-estimate the economic crises of advanced western societies, nevertheless the sense of certainty has gone and the belief that each generation will enjoy a higher standard of living than its predecessor is far less secure. Politics, too, in the west is possibly more abrasive than it was in the post-war decades and it certainly now breeds cynicism more easily than loyalty. And there would be few, if any, western societies that could claim a greater social cohesiveness as the millennium approaches. Even the image of science is tarnished as easy problems are solved but the intractable ones remain and the application of science creates problems of its own. But given the nature of the enemy that was conquered, even this scarcely seems to warrant the degree of pessimism that is now so frequently expressed.

Rather what has changed is the enemy itself. Like a creature from a contemporary animated children's television programme it has transformed itself into something quite different, and with a twist that bears a terrible irony, it is the solution that has become the problem. It is as if Superman, He-Man or She-Ra, instead of saving democracy and decency and putting to flight the forces of evil (with a little wit and a great deal of technology), have suddenly turned upon their adoring fans and proclaimed that there was nothing worth saving any more, that from now on they were going to do their own thing and to hell with the human race. As if Superman might explain his defection to Lois Lane by pointing out that it's not so much a question of the intellectual threat of new right ideology or the emotional blackmail of the moral majority, simply a question of survival in the modern world. Or as if She-Ra might whisper in the ear of Spirit, her flying unicorn, that it's hard being a women these days unless you have assertiveness training. Not that the high priests of modern social theory would put it quite like that. They would prefer to talk of the dilemmas of modernism, of the coming of postmodernism, of competing versions of feminism, of subjectivities and identities. But, however it might be expressed, the old enemy, industrialisation, has been replaced by the enemy within: modern society itself, with all its vaunted glories, has transformed itself before our eyes from hero to villain. The nuclear family, sitting down upon the sofa to watch their favourite television programme sees with horror an unfolding tale of narcissism in personal relationships; of intrusive technologies forcing people both into a narrow conformity through rampant consumerism; and at the same time, through the destruction of community, away from any real knowledge of each other's lived experiences.

Let us consider three plots they might encounter. To take first a not overly portentous issue, the brilliance of many contemporary picture books may lie not in anything so simple as the creator's empathy with children as was earlier suggested, but in their creators' ability to capture the postmodern, to play games with reality, to be metafictive, in short to exemplify the postmodern imagination (Lewis, 1990; Hunt, 1992; Moss, 1992). And in this sense, they do not celebrate childhood so much as present a disturbing picture of it; they offer, not simple representations of a world, but interpretations of it which play with reality, exploiting an imagination beyond the supposed simplicities of childhood's experience. A second plot, at the other end of the creative scale, tells of the commercialism that produces the imaginative desert of He-Man or She-Ra. This, as Kline has recently shown, is a plot in which sinister forces are at work. With the approval of the government of the most powerful nation in the world, forces operating within the toy and television industries exercise a control which is so overbearing, so immense and so adult that the child appears as nothing before it (Kline, 1993). Third, there is story that contains no trace of fiction. It is dominated by an image of the child in the last decade of the twentieth century, not cradled in the arms of a loving, confident parent, against a backdrop of caring school and wise professionals looking to the future, but of a murdered 2-year-old whose mangled body lies on a railway line in a decaying city on the north-west coast of a decaying country. It is of a child killed by his own kind, two boys who themselves had experienced, not an extremity of violence, but rather a dull, almost routine indifference and petty bullying (Miles, 1994). It was not the old enemy that seemed to haunt this tragedy, even though it was set against a post-industrial landscape, but rather modernity itself that had isolated a 2-year-old from his community even when he was amongst the shoppers in the precinct, and had separated his killers from ordinary human feelings when nobody had brutalised or starved them and nobody had forced them to live in the fetid squalor of a nineteenth-century slum. It is a sense of the impossibility of communication that will perhaps be the lasting memory: of the impossibility of communicating to distraught parents any coherent explanation beyond crude notions of evil and bestiality, and for ourselves, of wondering how this stark event can ever be rewritten to allow our precious conception of childhood innocence to survive (James and Jenks, 1994).

THE REPRESENTATION OF CRISIS

It is one thing to give an account of a late nineteenth-century moral panic about child prostitution, when a hundred years have anaesthetised its emotional impact and when historians have chewed over the facts of the case and offered a reasoned, distanced explanation. It is quite another to attempt the same with a situation in which one is living and participating. Nevertheless, it is important to try to analyse what elements make up the pervasive contemporary unease that surrounds the state of childhood. As James and Jenks point out in relation to the murder of James Bulger, there had been similar instances in the recent past, but on this occasion public perceptions seemed especially sensitive, reflecting a deep underlying anxiety. There was a sense of common ownership of guilt that grew out of the sheer incomprehension, but also out of the sense of its inevitability (James and Jenks, 1994). That sense of inevitability grew out of a long and complex process which had developed the sense of crisis over a period of two decades or more.

Any selection of material employed in recounting this narrative is bound to have an arbitrary element to it. Each separate strand develops a considerable literature of research and comment which is too extensive and diverse to summarise satisfactorily. Rather than attempt such a summary, it seems better to identify a small number of key texts to examine in more detail. Two general criteria have been employed in choosing these for discussion. One is that they should have a broad perspective which, consciously or unconsciously, intuitively or analytically, relates the specific to the general. Second, that there should be a sense of the emotions that underlie this crisis, since too distanced an approach leaves unspoken the anxiety that is so pervasive. This approach entails the use of texts where a clear attempt is being made to reach a broader audience since this is where these two criteria are most likely to be met. Such sources include the work of journalists and professional writers as well as mainstream academics, since the former represent a key mechanism in the articulation of this crisis.

Three broad areas have been chosen for this brief examination. One is the realm of the domestic, of the family and household. It is here that many have seen the decline of a key institution which supports supposedly traditional notions of childhood. Closely related to this is the perceived impact of changes in the role of women upon the family and its consequent effect upon children and the parent–child relationship especially. In this area, especially, the texts chosen do not represent a particular theoretical standpoint, nor are they necessarily those in which the use of empirical evidence meets the most rigorous standards. But they are amongst those that attempt to convey the crisis as an emotional whole to a wide audience, and as such they can indicate the nature of the contemporary discourse better than more traditional academic texts. The second area is that of the media and specifically the relationship between television and the state of childhood. Behind this lies a concern about the relationship of the child to adult knowledge and about the means by which access to that knowledge is controlled and regulated. The third area is the least tangible and relates to the way in which the sense of crisis about childhood is related to broader interpretations and theories about the nature of modern societies. The desire to theorise the crisis, to explain it in terms that relate to the broad movements of advanced western societies, produces both intuitive and highly schematic responses.

The child in the family

We won't, claims the advertisement of a British insurance company, make a drama out of a crisis. But in the world of social criticism the impetus towards theatricality is strong. In the early 1980s the American writer Marie Winn (probably best known for her book on television, *The Plug-In Drug* (1977)), published her *Children Without Childhood: Growing Up Too Fast in the World of Sex and Drugs* (1984). Her method is direct and simple: to talk to parents, children and child-professionals in a variety of geographical settings, to recount their stories and to add her own distinctive commentary, drawing upon literary and media sources to illustrate a point and, occasionally, to engage in debate. Shorn of the caveats, parentheses and abstractions of more conventional academic discourse, her message comes across in the form of a dramatic narrative, a story of the anxieties of middle-class America at the beginning of the Reagan era. Parents, she says, have lost control of their children; they, in turn, have lost their ability to be children as they increasingly inhabit a world that demands of them a precocity at odds with the very idea of childhood.

'Once upon a time,' she begins, warning us that this is a story that will strain our credulity, there was a story about a fictional girl called Lolita which was banned in Boston and reviled by the reviewer of the *New York Times*. But then, only a single generation later, Winn claims, and

> There is very little doubt that schoolchildren of the 1980s are more akin to Nabokov's nymphet than to those guileless and innocent creatures with their shiny Mary Janes and pigtails, their scraped knees and trusting ways that were called children not so long ago. . . . Something has happened to the joys of childhood.
>
> (Winn, 1984: 3)

Children are no longer protected, but are prepared for a harsh, over-sophisticated adult existence. They have lost the difference and specialness that used to be theirs as they are increasingly exposed to the 'secret underside' and 'hidden territories' of adult life. Nobody intended this, says Winn, nobody made a 'deliberate decision to treat kids in a new way'. Rather, 'it developed out of necessity. For children's lives are always a mirror of adult life' (ibid.: 5).

And the causes of this necessity?

> The great upheavals of the late 1960s and early 1970s – the so-called sexual revolution, the women's movement, the proliferation of television in American homes and its larger role in child rearing and family life, the rampant increase in divorce and single parenthood, political disillusionment in the Vietnam and post-Vietnam era, a deteriorating economic situation that propels more mothers into the work force – all these brought about changes in adult life that necessitated new ways of dealing with children.
>
> (ibid.: 5)

Of these many causes, we shall focus upon Winn's treatment of just two: the changing role of women and changes in family structure. Her account of the impact of the former goes under the title, 'The End of Symbiosis', and she refers directly to the nineteenth-century cult of femininity, and especially to the nature of the bond it established between women and children. The weakness of women in relation to men but their power over their offspring, she claims, led to children becoming 'the subjects of anxious care and protective nurture, the like of which had never been lavished on them before'. As women acquired particular qualities which marked them off from men, so children gained special attributes which 'they alone possessed – imaginativeness and playfulness', qualities which caused them to be treated differently from adults (ibid.: 113). For Winn, the consequences for the lives of women leaving the protective realm of the domestic are calamitous. Children could not be left behind in the domestic cocoon, but emerged with their mothers into the world of 'R-rated movies and live-in boyfriends and rape and murder and government corruption and all' (ibid.: 115). But as women themselves gained in authority and assertiveness and became more open about their frustrations, so they found it more difficult to be authoritative with their children. In challenging the patriarchal attitudes of their men, they lost their own traditional authority, encouraging in their children instead 'rudeness, disrespectfulness, open anger, whiny irritability, defiance' (ibid.: 116).

The more tangible consequences for women of their less childlike status, do not appear to Winn to bring advantages to children. Men and women, she believes, are frequently the gainers, but, without commensurate changes in the lives of men, children receive less care and supervision and consequently 'infiltrate adult life and find themselves partaking of adult experiences that they are developmentally unprepared to deal with' (ibid.: 122). Rising divorce rates and the consequent formation of complex households further force children away from their childhood to face the fallibility and insecurity of their parents, and in the absence of one parent, to take on the adult role of offering advice and even emotional support. Winn is sceptical of the rationalisation that children are better off out of an unhappy marriage. Such a belief, she claims, is based upon the growing assumption of shared interests between adults and children and a refusal to accept the separate needs of childhood.

Winn's defence of the state of childhood is based partly upon an acceptance of socio-biological interpretations of children's behaviour, but more upon the cultural need to prolong childhood in complex industrial societies. Latency may, she suggests, be imposed culturally to good effect in order to emphasise and extend those biologically determined childlike qualities of imaginativeness and playfulness. Even the repression of natural development may allow a positive intensification of these childhood abilities. Most significantly for Winn, only by having experienced a lengthy childhood, protected and nurtured by loving parents, can adults know sufficient of the needs of children to become successful parents themselves (ibid.: 203).

It is possible, of course, to take issue with Marie Winn upon many grounds. Her account is deliberately controversial, but it presents issues very much in the form in which they would be encountered by people, parents especially, in the course of their everyday lives – that is, in the context of a given 'here and now', largely unnegotiable. Its claims to authenticity come from the anecdotes of real people's lives and from the identification of their problems through popular culture, in contemporary films and novels. Academics and child-care professionals are brought in to support her argument, but the conviction comes more from the narrative she creates of the childhood's inexorable journey away from a Golden Age of Childhood (her own phrase) to a world in which survival depends upon a children's precocity, their ability to act the adult role with or without the necessary maturity or understanding.

Ten years after Marie Winn published *Children Without Childhood*, Rosalind Miles followed her studies of the contemporary state of women and of men by producing her account of the state of childhood in *The Children We Deserve*. Clearly two different authors writing in different contexts will produce different accounts, but two differences are striking and have perhaps a broader significance. The first lies in the emotional tone of the writing. Winn is combative and plain-speaking, but there is an underlying confidence that all is not lost, that if right-thinking people will but stand up and be counted good can yet prevail. The tone of Miles' writing is altogether more passionate but also more desperate, the calls for *something* to happen more insistent but less confident. The second difference is an ideological one. Winn is fairly happy with what is a frankly conservative agenda, albeit one dressed up in wholesome liberal sentiment. Miles would seem to present a more radical position in the sense that history appears to offer her nothing of value, but her radicalism leans heavily upon a therapeutic agenda for the establishment of personal identity and this gives an undeniably romantic gloss to her advocacy. Her dependence on the work of Alice Miller, for example, is very evident. Occasionally, though, the desperation breaks through, a sign perhaps of the growing frustrations that face the social critic of the late twentieth century. This is especially true of Miles who still believes in the possibility of human happiness, if only the young personality were not so damaged by having to live alongside other already mangled identities.

Miles' method is not dissimilar to that of Winn, but the techniques have become more sophisticated. This is the work of a writer familiar with the ways of the modern media. It is very much after the manner of the television documentary. The author provides a seamless narration which is expertly intercut with short, pithy, often emotionally charged quotations, ranging from official government statements and expert comment to a wide range of telling extracts from literary sources, especially poetry. These are interspersed with the anecdotal evidence of individuals to provide the vital element of authenticity, but unlike Winn, many of the cases cited in Miles' book are from interviews with media 'stars' (Roseanne Barr, Mia Farrow, Sinead O'Connor, etc.), culled from the weekend magazines of the broadsheets, figures whose stature within popular culture gives their personal experiences a special weight. And the whole is given gravity and weight by the constant reference to the expert. However, whilst Winn is not averse to cuffing an expert or two around the ear, Miles treats nearly all with great reverence – or at least those from the therapeutic stable. The object is not to engage in debate, but like the hard-hitting, campaigning television documentary, to build up layer upon layer of evidence and opinion in pursuit of one's cause.

So what is Miles' agenda? In essence it is a very simple one. The problem is that children have been neglected, not only individually, but by society as whole:

> For children in recent years have been getting an increasingly raw deal. From the Sixties revolt against authority which for the first time in history gave adults the right to become or remain children, to the emphasis of the Seventies on self-expression and self-discovery, through the 'Me-decade' of the Eighties on into the grim realism of the Nineties, *the pre-occupations of adults have dominated the agenda and the needs of children have been pushed to the back of the queue.*
>
> (Miles, 1994: xi; emphasis in original)

Children are clearly the victims and their advocates should join hands with feminists for the last great push for freedom:

> The rights of children must be the last frontier in the fight for freedom for us all, a consideration of their needs the last territory to be won back from the age-old tyranny of patriarchy and the casual brutality of its domination.
>
> (ibid.: x)

The problem, then, is in fact much older than the 1960s and more deep-seated than the narcissism attendant upon post-war affluence. Though Miles is principally concerned with the phenomenon of the here and now, she manages through this kind of rhetoric to suggest that the crisis of the late twentieth century has its origins buried deep in human history: 'Childhood has become a metaphor for a country that is out of control. The country hides its shame and self-hatred by regarding its young victims as culprits' (ibid.: 5).

In the late twentieth century, children have become victims of a pincer movement. On the one side is tradition, the cultural determinism that drives us to marry and have children because we know of no other way to spend our time. On the other is the destructive power of affluence and consumerism in which the child becomes an aspect of consumption and the 'designer child' the essential accessory to every successful partnership. As with Winn, but with less open acceptance, Miles has a sneaking respect for the 'old' family virtue of keeping marital conflicts and resentments hidden from the children. On the question of divorce, however, Miles has none of Winn's reticence: 'Can it be doubted any longer that *divorce is a form of child abuse*? . . . The parental assurance, 'it's better this way', provokes the child's protest of silent mutiny, '*not for me!*' (ibid.: 207; emphasis in original). The consequences for children in terms of single parenting, or increasingly for growing numbers of children of living in what Miles calls 'zero-parent families' where no biological parent is present, poses a 'challenge of nightmare proportions' (ibid.: 219).

Perhaps the biggest difference between Winn and Miles lies in the former's apparent lack of interest in child-abuse. 'Parent-battering' by children, it is true, gains a mention, but discussion of sexuality is concerned with teenage precocity not with abuse of children by adults. With Miles, ten years later, sexual abuse, and in particular its consistent under-reporting, represents the ultimate victimisation of children, a denial of their sense of individual identity, the final assault upon the defenceless by corrupt adult power. Furthermore, in the midst of uncertainties about what constitutes abuse, and about the possibility of False Memory Syndrome, the difficulties of bringing the problem into the light only serve to increase the sense of helplessness. For Miles, the core of this gnawing anxiety seems to be in the possibility that women themselves are abusers on a far greater scale than is commonly admitted. This is the 'question that the feminist movement prefers not to ask', the 'ultimate taboo' that surrounds this darkest of childhood nightmares (ibid.: 142). Not surprisingly, perhaps, it is a question that even Miles slides away from in pursuit of more visible aggressors. But to give voice to the fear at all is to raise the stakes even higher, since if mothers should fail their children in this way, what hope is left?

In Miles' grim vision, the designer baby adored in its cradle passes through a world bent upon conspicuous consumption, through broken families and anonymous unstable households, endures abuse and indifference, and emerges to be the victim who turns upon society in its incoherent rage. Children have become in the 1990s, says Beatrix Campbell, 'the enemy within . . . the pariahs who patrolled political discourse, producing panic wherever they went sniffing or stealing or suffering' (quoted ibid.: 251). Their loss is the loss of the self; in the words of Sinead O'Connor of 'My own inner child/Who is really me' (quoted ibid.: 242). It is this commitment to the idea of the self, to some core or essence which has to hold together to make an integrated human being (this 'inner-child racket' as one of O'Connor's critics put it), which seems most to affect Miles. That apart, her solutions are somewhat banal, as in all fairness most solutions inevitably tend to be, but that romance of the self, the belief in the soul as the seat of the well-adjusted, autonomous individual, is characteristic of much radical contemporary thinking. And when applied to the child with the urgency and passion of a writer like Miles it raises the emotional temperature and feeds the sense of crisis. It becomes not the relatively simple question of what are we to do, but the unanswerable one of what are we to be?

Not all writers feel the need to deal in such an emotional way with the contemporary state of childhood. The journalist and programme maker, Mukti Jain Campion is altogether more brisk. Her book, *Who's Fit to be a Parent?*, has a narrower scope than either Winn or Miles and is much more concerned with the relationship between the law, child-professionals and the increasing variety of household and family forms in which parenting takes place. Her method is as sophisticated as Miles', but is more akin to radio documentary than television. More conventional academic sources are employed, the emotional tug of the carefully placed quotation is eschewed, and there is a strand of sinewy argumentativeness that runs throughout the whole book. But, for all her briskness, Campion is not insensitive to the historical moment:

> We have reached a dramatic point in the history of children's rights in relationship to their parents, and the way forward is littered with

> ambiguities and dangers which we need to address. What does society want for children and what does it expect from parents?
> (Campion, 1995: 2)

There is much more acceptance of, and indeed a welcome for, some of the trends in household formation, and an enthusiasm for varieties of parenting which would have caused much greater concern to either Winn or Miles. In particular, Campion is more positive about the possibilities of children surviving the experience of divorce or single parenting. Her concern in this, as in questions of child abuse, is that the state and its agencies should provide a satisfactory framework, within which disputes can be quickly settled and allegations of abuse investigated.

In contrast to Winn, who tends to look back on the 1950s as a golden age, Campion is critical of the traditional image of the family with its 'closed belief systems' and oppressive paternalism, and unlike Miles she wants nothing of the psychoanalytical approaches that in her view were also one of the sins of the 1950s (ibid.: 278). The cultural diversity of the late twentieth century requires other methods, she claims. She opposes an Ideal and an Actual model of parenting, the former representing the alleged ideals of the 1950s, the latter the reality of the 1990s. Words such as 'duty, obligation, conformity' are replaced with 'needs, rights and personal choice'. In establishing the criteria for fit parenting, what matters is not what you are but what you do, and 'parenting' as a definable activity replaces 'parents' who by mere accident of nature, it would seem, have in the past been left to look after their biological offspring. And as parents increasingly see their role in terms of a job, so parenting becomes more like managing, and thus a suitable case for the application of management theory. Total Quality Management, one of the glories of contemporary management theory, comes like a modern knight in very shiny armour to facilitate the development of skills that will enable the parent to 'address any problem that arises independently and effectively'. What we need to do, claims Campion with practised lack of emotion, is to stop sentimentalising children and prevent charities, in their advertising campaigns, from using 'pathetic pictures of abused or neglected children'. We should look rather to children's future role, their coming duties and expectations, their importance to our future welfare:

> At present they seem to serve no useful purpose other than (possibly) to bring their parents some emotional reward and so charities can appeal to people's pity. Society needs to be reminded

> of the value of children. It can then be more clear-headed about what it requires parenting to achieve.
>
> (ibid.: 288)

This is advocacy for the final obliteration of the public/private distinction and for bringing children firmly into the public domain through the rationalism of modern management theory. From there it is a short step to giving parenting the final accolade, a state licence, though Campion stops (only just) short of this final endorsement.

For all three writers discussed here, there is a crisis in the modern family which has profound effects upon the state of childhood, but which academic research finds it difficult to shed light on. The demographics of household composition, to take just one example, are extremely complex, both in understanding the patterns of the past and even in tracing, let alone interpreting, contemporary trends. Qvortrup, for example, has pointed out that much routine demographic data is not collected in a form that allows us to explore its impact upon the experience of the child. It provides snapshots which do not necessarily illuminate the dynamics of household formation which are vital to any assessment of children's actual experience; children, he claims, have no 'voice' in social accounting (Qvortrup, 1990, 1991). Comparisons with historical patterns, too, are frequently naive. Suggesting, for example, that the complex families caused by parental death and remarriage are comparable with the considerably more complex households and family relationships caused by divorce and remarriage, is to trivialise the child's experience on the basis of snap-shot pictures of household compositions across time. Research into the effects on children of divorce is, not surprisingly, inconclusive (Miles and Campion can confidently draw differing conclusions), and the whole complex of issues surrounding child abuse, and sexual abuse in particular, threatens to send the debate spiralling across the social landscape with all the destructive power of a tornado (Stainton Rogers, 1992; Kincaid, 1992). Even the potentially calming sociological voice that seems genuinely to be searching for ways of letting children speak of their own lives and preoccupations will find it difficult to compete with the anguished cries of Miles' psychotherapists or with the brash conviction of Campion's management theorists (Mayall, 1994; Brannen and O'Brien, 1995a, b).

But the issues surrounding childhood are, as they were a hundred years ago, foremost on the social agenda and therefore the writing, the investigation, the comment and the argument will continue. What in

Stead's day was a relatively parochial political skirmish confined very largely to the capital city (W.H. Smith refused to sell *The Pall Mall Gazette* at the time of the Eliza Armstrong case) has now global dimensions, and the methodologies and techniques for investigation and media exploitation are infinitely greater. In such a climate the conditions for creating a sense of crisis are ideal. This is not to suggest in any way that writers like Winn, Miles and Campion are not serious in their anxieties or in the proposals they make for remedying the situation; they are all more knowledgable, scrupulous and committed than ever W.T. Stead was. Certainly, their audience is predominantly amongst the chattering classes, but then that is true (given a tolerant definition of social groups) for most of the material presented in this book. What is important to grasp about such commentaries is that they do speak of a social crisis. To what extent that crisis exists at the level of children's experience, and whether in any summative sense that is a better or worse experience than that of a child of the Victorian lower middle classes or of a Puritan yeoman family of the 1640s, we shall never know. Rather the stories they tell have to be understood as commentaries upon the anxieties, neuroses, hopes and fears of our own society.

Childhood in the television age

If the apparent disruption of the domestic scene is one source of the contemporary sense of crisis, then the impact of television and more recently of video and computers upon the state of childhood is undoubtedly another. Once again the potential literature is vast, ranging from studies which attempt, inconclusively, to establish the 'effect' of television upon children's behaviour, to those which attempt through semiotics and audience research to explore television literacy and the social context in which viewing takes place (Gunter and McAleer, 1990; van Evra 1990; Hodge and Tripp, 1986; Buckingham, 1993a, b). However, two books stand out as having attempted to place the issue of children and television in a broader historical context and as seeing in the late twentieth-century situation something which threatens the state of childhood itself. These are Neil Postman's *The Disappearance of Childhood* (1983) and Stephen Kline's *Out of the Garden: Toys, TV and Children's Culture in the Age of Marketing* (1993).

Postman's book was first published in the early 1980s at much the same time as Winn's *Children Without Childhood*, which also identified television as a major cause of the erosion of childhood's special status. A little earlier David Elkind had published his study of precocity in contemporary childhood, *The Hurried Child* (1981). Education, suggests Elkind, extends our memory by transmitting a cultural past, but the media extend our senses, and television especially 'removes many of the intellectual barriers other media put in the way of accessing information' (ibid.: 75). Furthermore, the accessibility of information via television breaks up the rigid age-stratification so carefully developed in western education systems, thus eroding distinctions within childhood itself. Some of these ideas were developed by Meyrowitz, Postman's student in the 1970s, who explored the impact of electronic media upon the process of socialisation and in particular the shift from literary to oral and visual communications media:

> Reading and writing involve an abstract code of arbitrary and semantically meaningless symbols. To read and write efficiently, these symbols must be memorized, practised and internalized. The complexity of the print's code excludes very young children from virtually all communications in print. . . . The varying complexity of the code in print not only serves to isolate children from adult situations, but works as well to isolate adults from children's situations.
>
> (Meyrowitz, 1984: 30)

Television, on the other hand, with its iconic signs and human voices, needs no access to these complex, abstract decoding skills, and therefore access to its information cannot be controlled by the many devices adults have designed to monitor children's access to printed material. The problem lies in the nature of the medium itself:

> Contrary to many claims . . . children's access to adult information through television is not simply the result of a lapse in parental authority and responsibility. Print provides many filters and controls that television by its very nature cannot. No matter what parents do, short of removing the television set altogether, the old information environment cannot be fully reinstated. And even if the set is removed from one child's home, there are certainly sets in the homes of friends and relatives.
>
> (ibid.: 35)

Meyrowitz goes on to sketch a thesis suggesting that the concept of childhood innocence was tied closely to the age of print media, when adults could control access to the burgeoning quantity of information that flowed from the invention of the printing press. Literacy became a critical prerequisite of full adult status (something that the lower classes and women were also to learn), and in the case of children especially, innocence became a state defined as one without adult knowledge.

In his elaboration and popularisation of some of these ideas, Postman focuses upon the concept of shame, arguing that 'without a well-developed idea of shame, childhood cannot exist' (Postman, 1983: 9). Provocatively, Postman contrasts Erasmus's Colloquies of the early sixteenth century, concerned with teaching boys how to 'regulate their instinctual life', with the children's fiction of the contemporary American writer, Judy Blume, who deals frankly with teenage sexuality. Erasmus, Postman observes, was in some sense the Judy Blume of his day, but he was concerned to increase a sense of shame, Blume to reduce it (ibid.: 48). With the coming of the television age, for the reasons Meyrowitz adduces, childhood innocence is lost and 'the idea of shame diluted and demystified' (ibid.: 85). Arguing from the ideas of Freud and Norbert Elias, Postman suggests that the civilising process, the belief that civilisation cannot exist without the control of natural instincts, goes into reverse. It is the hiding from public view, the rendering of adult instincts mysterious, that allows the civilised society to regulate them and to control the access of children to the knowledge associated with them. Thus, before the advent of television,

> Children . . . are immersed in a world of secrets, surrounded by mystery and awe; a world that will be made intelligible to them by adults who will teach them, in stages, how shame is transformed into a set of moral directives. From the child's point of view, shame gives power and authority to adulthood. For adults know, whereas children do not, what words are shameful to use, what subjects are shameful to discuss, what acts are deemed necessary to privatise.
>
> (ibid.: 86)

But television destroys this adult control over what is shameful, as sexuality, aggression and the many, varied problems of modern societies are made visible to the child through the 'total disclosure medium'. It is not, argues Postman, that questions surrounding death, mental illness, homosexuality should remain 'dark and mysterious secrets' as the 'Moral Majority' might wish, it is rather that through television, adults lose control of when and how such matters come to the attention of children.

> For if there are no dark and fugitive mysteries for adults to conceal from children, and then to reveal to them as they think necessary, safe, and proper, then surely the dividing line between adults and children becomes dangerously thin . . . it is clear that if we turn over to children a vast store of powerful adult material, childhood cannot survive. By definition adulthood means mysteries solved and secrets uncovered. If from the start children know the mysteries and the secrets, how shall we tell them apart from anyone else?
>
> (ibid.: 88)

Having established the primary cause of the disappearance of childhood firmly within the realm of communications technology, Postman then goes on to list the consequences. The sexualisation of the child in popular culture is epitomised for Postman in the shift from Shirley Temple to Brooke Shields and from Walt Disney's children to those of Judy Blume. On television itself, the game show epitomises the growth of the 'adultified' child illustrating the process of convergence between child and adult:

> a game show is a parody of sorts of a classroom in which contestants are duly rewarded for obedience and precociousness but are otherwise subjugated to all the indignities that are traditionally the schoolchild's burden.
>
> (ibid.: 127)

More and more children become central figures in soap opera, their preoccupations merging with those of adults. Even children's games are either disappearing or are being organised and packaged increasingly by adults. Increased juvenile crime, teenage pregnancies, sexually transmitted diseases, alcohol and drug abuse, rising divorce rates, the growth of child liberationist movements – all these are related in some way to the disappearance of the concept of childhood brought about by the coming of television and the decline of adult control through traditional literacy. To resist these effects, Postman claims, now means,

> conceiving of parenting as an act of rebellion against American culture . . . to insist that one's children learn the discipline of delayed gratification, or modesty in their sexuality, or self-restraint

> in manners, language and style is to place oneself in opposition to almost every social trend.... But most rebellious of all is the attempt to control the media's access to one's children.
>
> (ibid.: 153)

As with the writings of Winn and Miles, much of what Postman has to say is often deliberately contentious and tendentious. Such an approach lays the writer inevitably open to criticisms coming from a wide range of perspectives. In particular, with some degree of variation, all three writers are consciously trying to steer a difficult path between, on the one hand, what they see as the need to publicise the increasing dangers for childhood in contemporary society and, on the other, a desire not to be categorised as reactionary, anti-feminist, part of the American 'Moral Majority' or as simply wallowing in nostalgia. Postman, in particular, with a personal biography as an American radical, is anxious to keep his distance from simple conservatism, though he is astute enough to know when it can be used as a stick with which to beat a flabby liberalism (ibid.: 148). Hence it is not only the content of their writing that is significant but also the way their quite complex positional manoeuvring sheds light on the interweaving discourses (about the future of the family, the role of women, the impact of television, consumerism and popular culture, for example), all of which have implications for childhood in the late twentieth century. What in a sense they are trying to do is to abstract childhood from the complex of ideological, social and economic forces that shape it, and to give it an independent voice. Whilst they are acutely aware of the dependent and determined nature of childhood, they strive to give the child a voice alongside that of women, and against consumerism and the mass media. In so doing, they have to generate, not simply intellectual arguments which are always going to be open to counter-argument, but also the emotional atmosphere that is essential to generating the appropriate sense of crisis. It is as much in this sense as any other that they constitute important texts, illustrative of the discursive battles that influence parenting, education, social policy and the regulatory interface between society and capitalism in the late twentieth century.

Regulating the capitalism–consumer interface – the case of toys and television

It was the Victorians who taught us how to surround childhood with emotion and how to generate a politics of social reform that depended at least as much upon feeling as it did upon intellectual rigour. In the late twentieth century, however, even though the skills of the crisis makers have been developed, they address a more cynical audience, one more used to distancing itself from emotional appeals. Even more importantly, however, they now face important economic interests, as powerful perhaps as those of the early nineteenth-century factory owners who opposed the regulation of child labour, but infinitely more subtle and insidious. If the early nineteenth-century argument was about the role of children as producers, in the late twentieth century it has become increasingly concerned with their role as consumers. Stephen Kline's study of the impact of the marketing of children's toys through television on children's culture is perhaps one of the most significant studies of contemporary consumerism (Kline, 1993). Kline's is a substantial study in a traditional academic mould and draws upon important research data as well as offering theoretically sophisticated frameworks within which to interpret it. It belongs to the literature being discussed in this chapter, however, because it depends upon the sense of crisis to speak to a wider audience; certainly the British media have identified him as a spokesperson on consumerism and children's culture (for example, BBC, 1994). Kline also engages with the widespread unease about television and children and, though his response is measured and careful, the engagement is avowedly that of parent as well as academic, and the challenge to economic interests is direct and unequivocal.

Kline's thesis rests upon the proposition that 'the expanding scale of marketing to children represents a powerful but ambiguous vector in our children's lives' (Kline, 1993: viii). He challenges the view that socialisation rests with the family and school: 'There is also an invisible hand in the market, which influences childhood by shaping the things children use and the media through which they learn about them' (ibid.: 19). We know too little, he argues, about the way in which what children learn through media representation (whether it be literary or televisual) is incorporated into their cognitive development, and into the way they interpret the world around them. We know that play is central to this process but understand it very little.

He notes, as do so many others, that studies of the impact of television upon children's behaviour are inconclusive and ambiguous, but that may be, he suggests, because we are naive in seeking direct, measurable cause and effect mechanisms. He refers with approval to Postman's study and to the way it draws attention to the technologies of communication, but drawing upon the work of Raymond Williams, he is critical of the assumption that 'the patterns of its use and meaning . . . were inherent in the technology itself' (ibid.: 71). It is, as Williams argues, in the social relations of production and consumption, in the dynamics of cultural production not in technology alone, that influences are shaped. Kline is also critical of Postman's emphasis upon the areas in which adult and child culture tend to merge – those areas of popular culture (especially film and television) which older children and adults increasingly share. This is to neglect, argues Kline, the important impact of consumerism upon children's culture itself. It is not just that children are increasingly drawn into adult patterns of consumption, but also that in their own world of children's play the interference of the invisible (adult) hand of capitalism is ever more important:

> from the early 1950s television producers became engaged in developing a new kind of television product with a very different sensibility and imagery at its core. These creations were first shown after school, later on Saturday mornings, and later still in the preschool hours, whenever children could be drawn to the set without the parent in the room . . . television has become the undisputed leader in the production of children's culture.
>
> (ibid.: 73)

Kline's focus is upon developments in American children's television especially during the period of deregulation in the 1980s. It is of course true that, in Britain, television is a more controlled medium and that children's television still holds a special place, legally endorsed at least in terrestrial television. Even in Britain, however, deregulation remains on the political agenda, and the BBC itself, even with its long tradition of special children's programming, is increasingly under intense financial pressure (Blumler, 1992). The developments which Kline describes taking place in the United States have relevance for the rest of the western world; no western society remains immune from the forces which are the subject of his discussion.

The production of commercial children's television became dependent upon the advertisers' desire to use children's programming in order to gain access to the growing children's market. Before the spread of television, children had remained somewhat inaccessible to advertising, but television opened up the possibility of speaking to children of their wants and fantasies without adult mediation. Seeing the potential of addressing their advertisements directly to children, the makers of toys and games invested heavily in research that would tell them how to achieve their objectives most effectively. Out of this investment by the marketing industry in the playing and viewing habits of children emerged the promotional toy, the character tied in with a particular product. Speaking directly to children, it was less necessary to persuade parents that toys had an educational value; all that was needed was for them to tie in with the animated cartoons that had become the predominant form of production for children's television. As a consequence, in the freer, deregulated climate of the Reagan presidency, the animated cartoon featuring characters that could be bought as toys in the shops became the staple diet of children's television production with the consequence that 'the rise in character marketing has all but eliminated images of real children playing in the normal course of their lives – in dramas or narratives about and for the young' (ibid.: 141).

Thus both the nature of toys and the nature of television were changed by the marketing needs of consumer capitalism, and children were 'catapulted into a fantastic and chaotic time–space continuum of action toys' (ibid.: 140). Or rather the boys were, because for girls there was Barbie and My Little Pony and the Care Bears. One of the most dramatic consequences of these developments, according to Kline, is the rigid sex-stereotyping that comes in their wake. Market researchers found that children's play was strongly gender determined with little cross-over of toys, and manufacturers responded accordingly producing a precisely segregated market (ibid.: 195, 245ff, 306ff).

Parents, too, are drawn into encouraging the consumerism of their children by the feeling that part of the process of growing up involves learning how to be a consumer, of having money to spend and learning how to make decisions about how to spend it. Through consumption, too, the child learns the importance of lifestyle; of establishing identity, not through occupation or social role, but through elaborate patterns of consumption. The development of shopping as a leisure activity made consumerism a family activity that could also involve the children. The marketers noticed too that changes in household patterns and in the affluence of the retired could be usefully exploited. Divorced parents visiting their children would be inclined to bring presents, as perhaps would those working long hours and with less time to spend with their children. Grandparents too, increasingly affluent but perhaps less directly involved with their grandchildren, might also be inclined to use the toy as a way of maintaining a relationship (ibid.: 179ff).

However difficult it may be to be precise about the effects of these developments upon children's attitudes, behaviour and capacities, Kline's is a sober assessment. The synergy created between toys and television, he suggests, 'induces a unique mode of consciousness' in which watching television has become 'a primer for learning the particular mental prerequisites of character play' (ibid.: 323). The narrative, imaginative and moral limitations of television geared primarily to the needs of the market that can be witnessed in He-Man, Care Bears or a host of other programmes cannot but affect children's play adversely, claims Kline. Though the conclusions he draws from his own research are cautious, 'Yet', he comments, 'we cannot help feeling as we watch these children at play that their activities are sex-typed, stereotypic and predictable' (ibid.: 331). Parents are excluded from involvement in their children's play, and the play itself becomes ever more remote from real human experience:

> The abstract and alienated thematics of character fiction means that children are unlikely to play out with these toys fantasy scenes of going to school, being ill or waking up frightened, still less peer rejection or the death of a pet. It's not impossible, of course, but they simply don't interpret their toys in that way. And this means that the potential to schematize and master in play a whole range of difficult emotional material is also absent in their lives.
>
> (ibid.: 335)

It would be possible to interpret Kline as presenting arguments which contradict those of Winn and Postman especially. After all he expresses anxieties about the exclusion of children from the adult world, not their over-exposure to it. Part of the reason for this lies in the different age ranges that preoccupy the different writers; Kline's focus is more specifically upon quite young children who play with toys rather than play at crime or sex. But at a deeper level he seems to reinforce their concerns. The nature of children's play is certainly an important aspect of Kline's work, but his overriding preoccupation is with the impact of consumer capitalism upon the childhood experience:

> Children are simply finding their place within our consumer culture. But does this constitute a harm to children or diminish or interfere with their maturation? Clearly not, for these children are simply being socialized into the way of life of our consumer culture.
>
> (ibid.: 349)

This is as bleak a conclusion as any of the more horrific, sensational ones drawn by Miles. Those who sell toys and television will claim that they give children what they want (and take far more care over finding out what children want than most), and that they do them no harm (or at least no harm that can be positively identified). But why, demands Kline, should we allow the marketplace so much influence over the socialisation of our children, why should we abandon them to the adult world of consumerism, of the marketer, the toy manufacturer and the television executive? Economics is not separate from culture and the invisible hand of the market has nothing intelligent to say about the social, moral or emotional criteria that should shape the response of parents, teachers or indeed the media to the responsibility of overseeing the growth of the next generation.

Theorising the crisis

There is much to be said for leaving the discussion at this stage, with that combination of emotional commitment, more or less systematically collected evidence, and (at least in Kline's case) a clearly and strongly argued analysis. The 'value added' to be gained by venturing further into the realms of social theory is frankly uncertain. As Rex and Wendy Stainton Rogers have shown, if rather self-consciously, there is much fun as well as a great deal of insight to be gained from the unleashing of postmodernist methodologies upon the stories we tell of the nature of childhood (Stainton Rogers, 1992). But they had seen the postmodernist light on their personal road to Damascus and had the specific discipline of developmental psychology to convert: that kind of theoretical play needs an opponent of some kind. In any case this present study is tied to an older agenda in which we seek for some meta-narrative that 'explains' the contemporary state of childhood in terms of the history of the west. In this respect, the contribution of the Stainton Rogers' is clear. Science has given to the west a perception of children as a problem which science can solve, especially when science is helped by a politics of social reform which clearly identifies heroes and villains. Such 'modernist moral analyses' are not liked by the Stainton Rogers, whether they be of the kind that, like some feminisms, constitute men as the villains whilst ignoring the many conflicts of interest between woman and children, or of the kind that rummages for enemies in the dustbins of individual or social pathologies:

> This kind of endeavour implies (when it does not explicitly claim) a credulous and singularised utopianism – that all that needs to be done 'to stamp out the problem' is to overthrow the patriarchy, or remove violence from television, or disband the social work profession, or liberate children from the shackles of adult power – and all our problems will be solved! Child concern thus becomes reconstituted as a moral crusade, not just by populist politicians and the press, but by the vast majority of practitioners, scholars and those who see themselves as advocates for the child.
>
> (Stainton Rogers, 1992: 190)

Of course they are right. It is all very well for Winn and Miles to berate the contemporary family, for Postman to see a conspiracy in a piece of electronic equipment and for Kline to despair at our indifference to capitalism's infiltration of children's culture, but these are only preludes to the campaigns which must inevitably follow – for licensed parenting, for a more protective schooling and for a better regulated media. But before the campaigns begin, there are questions which lurk around the edges of the writings discussed in this chapter which are not entirely answered by ascribing to modernist 'analytics', as the Stainton Rogers call them, the principal role in the contemporary crisis of childhood, significant though they may be.

In their discussion of the modern family Brigitte and Peter Berger attempt an interpretation in an old-fashioned meta-narrative style. Modernisation theory, they suggest, might yet offer some explanation both of the historically changing role of the family through its complex interactions with the development of modern capitalist industrial societies, and also of its contemporary, ambiguous state within the modern social order. Emphasising the role of consciousness in social change rather than that of institutions, the Bergers point to Weber's conception of rationalisation as one which might help to explain the long process of adaptation the family has made in its journey through modern society. And alongside this they point to a growing consciousness about the importance of individualism and individual privacy (Berger and Berger, 1983: 85ff). The history they present is one in which child-rearing practices are increasingly shaped by a consciousness in which rationality and a belief in individualism become ever more significant.

This kind of sociologist's history is now with good reason somewhat unfashionable, relying as it does so heavily upon grand conceptual analysis to bear the weight of an over-generalised empirical analysis. Nevertheless the grand concept is not without value, and Berger and Berger explore theirs with some energy. Rationalism and individualism they define as follows:

> Rationalism refers to a mind-set orientated towards *control* – to wit, towards controlling the world by rational calculation. And individualism refers to both the belief in and the psychological reality of *autonomy* – to wit, an attitude on the part of the individual of independence, self-assertion, and if necessary dissent *vis-à-vis* society.
>
> (ibid.: 109)

In terms of child-rearing this means producing 'individuals with "character"' and for Berger and Berger this is the ultimate aim of the ideal bourgeois family – the production of male children especially, for whom individualism is located in 'character', and whose strength of character determines their response to the demands of society through the exercise of conscience. Such a process of child-rearing required detailed planning and execution, becoming the primary duty of the bourgeois family. It depended critically upon the achievement of a balance 'between individualism and social responsibility, between "liberation" and strong communal ties, between acquisitiveness and altruism' (ibid.: 117).

This important balance was always difficult to achieve and precarious to maintain. What supported it, claim Berger and Berger, was religion, and Protestantism in particular, operating as a 'higher force, located outside the individual, the family, and society as a whole'. With the advance of secularisation 'the religious underpinnings of the bourgeois balancing act weakened and the earlier unity of values came to be polarised into antagonistic alternatives' (ibid.: 117). Consequently rationality and individualism turn, in the modern consciousness, into hyper-rationality and hyper-individualism as the family moves not to postmodernity but to hyper-modernity. An 'engineering mentality' determines notions of a normal childhood or good parenting which, when applied to actual life, 'become *cliches*, mindlessly mouthed as "recipe knowledge" . . . and in consequence the most intimate human relationships – between spouses and children, above all – acquire a strange patina of abstraction' (ibid.: 119). Individualism also becomes radicalised and 'the search for individual identity in isolation from all communal definitions becomes a central concern of life' supported by the idea that 'socialisation distorts an originally positive human nature, which can be freed from the unnatural constraints imposed on it by society' (ibid.: 120).

A not dissimilar interpretation is to be found in the work of Basil Bernstein on cultural reproduction. In his famous discussion of the modern British infant school, he bases his analysis upon a distinction that he draws between the culture of the old (middle) class, founded upon a conception of 'individuation', and that of the new class (the 'regulators, repairers, diffusers, shapers and executors' of cultural reproduction), founded upon a conception of 'personalised' differentiation. Central to his theory is a contrast between the concepts of the 'individual' and of the 'person':

> Whereas the concept of the individual leads to specific, unambiguous role identities and relatively inflexible role performances, the concept of the person leads to ambiguous personal identity and flexible role performances.
>
> (Bernstein, 1977: 125)

Elaborating upon this notion, we might say that there are two competing discourses each claiming to know how best to shape the next generation. For the old class, cultural reproduction is based upon rules which are made explicit to the children themselves, rules concerned with hierarchy, the sequencing of knowledge and the evaluative criteria employed in assessment of all kinds of learning. And at a more general level, the intention is to locate the subject (the individual identity) appropriately within a strictly defined range of role possibilities. Thus, for example, in relation to class, gender and even personality clichés (pretty, clever, reliable, brave, etc.), the individual is, through a clear sequence of developments, located and evaluated in relation to pre-existing models. In the discourses of the new class, on the other hand, there is a conception of self, of identity, being inherent in the newborn child, of a soul that needs freedom to develop in its own terms, of a concept of biologically determined development which must take its own natural course. To confront the child with pre-existing forms is to threaten deformation of the personality. Hence all the rules of cultural reproduction (though they cannot be dispensed with) are hidden and remain undisclosed to the child.

In Bernstein's own discussion, the infant school has become the domain of the new class through the propagation of the 'invisible pedagogy', through which professionals exercise a discreet but intense surveillance over the children who learn through play. These professionals antagonise the parents of both the old class and the working class who still expect explicit rules to govern the transmission of culture. Notions of the ordering of time, of the regulation of space and of the mechanisms of social control are, in the invisible pedagogy, less explicit but more complex, and the language in which they are articulated more elaborate. The child (unknowingly) and the professional (with expert knowledge of the child's innate propensities) enter into a complex, apparently non-hierarchical, non-evaluative relationship which steers the child towards its own unique destiny.

For all the difference in focus and in context, there are possible connections here between Bernstein and Berger and Berger. The latter's notions of hyper-rationalism and hyper-individualism find echoes in Bernstein's invisible pedagogy. In the concept of the person is a kind of hyper-individualism, a desire for the individual identity to be free of constraint and a rejection of stereotypical role performance. But there is also a sense of hyper-rationality in the complexity of the 'hidden' rules of cultural transmission of the invisible pedagogy, a process which Bernstein insists exposes more of the individual child to the gaze of the teacher than the older 'visible pedagogy' ever did. Thus the radicalisation of socialisation becomes a contradictory exercise, just as it does for Berger and Berger, offering apparently greater freedom through a free-floating individualism but at the same time controlling through a complex surveillance system heavily dependent upon what the Stainton Rogers would no doubt dismiss as a particularly nasty form of modernising 'analytics'. This contradiction is in fact perfectly captured, albeit unawares, by Rosalind Miles, who longs for the child to be free of the gross interference of parents, but who nevertheless demands from them firm parenting. Miles, too, exhibits in her writing a dependence upon the psychology and psychotherapy industry which is so despised by the Stainton Rogers, criticised by the Bergers as covering parent–child interactions with that 'strange patina of abstraction' and, by implication, identified by Bernstein as a priestly voice behind the invisible pedagogy.

The political scientist, Dillon, once described a 'disciplinary matrix' within which decisions are made in modern political systems, a matrix of beliefs in the power of reason which in the process of real decision-making comes face to face with an irrational and unpredictable reality – a 'precarious experience', he calls it. In such a situation, the decision-maker faces both constant failure and constant demands to avoid failure through ever more rational action. The result is that political responses become ever more dramaturgical, pieces of theatre which attempt to disguise an impossible conflict. Dramaturgy, Dillon says, refers to 'a pre-occupation with generating and employing symbolic and stylised representations of form (or reality) so as to propagate or sustain a given intellectual, organisational or social order' (Dillon, 1976: 55). The policy maker,

> mediates . . . between precarious experience and the social order which depends upon a disciplinary matrix to bind it together. To do this he must employ dramatic and symbolic devices to represent the consistency and sense of purpose in his actions.
>
> (ibid.: 58)

If for policy maker we substitute parent, or teacher, or child-professional or even writer of books about the state of childhood in the late twentieth century, then Dillon's acute observations upon the policy making process suggest a wider application. For if, as the Bergers suggest, the modern consciousness, both within and about the family, has become 'hyper' (enters, in Dillon's terms, the disciplinary matrix of rationality), then responses to its problems will inevitably acquire a dramaturgical quality. Bernstein, albeit focusing on the specific context of education, also suggests a more general unease and ambiguity surrounding the process of cultural transmission. And whilst his analysis is closely tied in to an analysis of a fracturing middle class, he identifies the consequent tensions as having implications beyond that fraction of the middle class where the invisible pedagogy arises. In his description of the invisible pedagogy, there is a clear sense of a strategy that over-reaches itself, of one that pushes too hard to be rational and places an unrealistic burden upon the shaper (teacher, parent) and shaped (child) in their pursuit of individual identity.

Nor should we be surprised if emotion is as significant in the theatrical experience as are more cerebral elements. The Stainton Rogers complain that 'We have not so much got the means to tackle child concern as an emotional market *in* child concern' (Stainton Rogers, 1992: 195; emphasis in original). And again, of course, they are right. Any explanation of the nature of the discourse of crisis surrounding childhood has to take account of this emotionality as inherent in the 'hyper' state of consciousness that the Bergers describe, with its attendant 'analytics', its 'invisible pedagogies' and its 'dramaturgies'.

The texts examined earlier in this chapter, those of Winn, Miles, Campion, Postman and even to some extent Kline, both reflect upon and themselves reflect hyper-modernity. They are intensely critical of its impact upon the family and upon the process of socialisation and cultural transmission, particularly its encouragement of narcissistic forms of individualism, Bergers' hyper-individualism, which Winn and Miles especially believe now dominate the family. They also fear the impact of consumer capitalism as a force which takes away parental and even teacher control over the construction of identity and, as Kline especially argues, hands over the business of cultural transmission to the economics of the marketplace. But they also reflect in different ways what the Bergers see as the other half of the problem, hyper-rationality. Winn, in a sense, is the least affected because hers is the most conservative response and ends only with a nostalgic longing for that which is gone, but Miles, with her reliance upon the psychotherapeutic agenda, and Campion, with her belief in the latest management theory, very clearly illustrate the dramaturgical response. Even Postman and Kline reveal a dependence upon 'analytics', a belief that to analyse the problem is to begin to solve it. Though to be fair, Postman honestly acknowledges his bafflement as to what solutions there might be.

This has been a brief and frankly eclectic search for some more general explanation of the contemporary crisis believed by so many to be facing childhood in contemporary western societies. The Bergers' conceptions of hyper-rationalism and hyper-individualism have an ad hoc, almost home-spun quality to them which does not necessarily detract from their usefulness. Nevertheless, theory does like to belong to some broader strain of thought and to present a tidier face to the world. It will be evident to those with an interest in such matters that what has been discussed here pulls in the direction of interpretations that speak of the postmodern. The Stainton Rogers use it as a methodological device rather than as a theory, and Bernstein is still tied to class-related explanations, but the clear Weberianism of the Bergers, their interpretation of history through modernisation theory and their emphasis upon rationalism and individual identity, inevitably draw one towards explanations which emphasise the postmodern condition. Complex and elaborate as these explanations are, the work of Jenks provides a neat and accessible entry to them whilst not losing sight of our central focus upon the state of childhood (Jenks, 1994).

Jenks sets out to explore the contemporary anguish over child abuse and finds an explanation within accounts of the postmodern condition. He argues that the rise in documented cases of child abuse needs to be explained in terms of the wider condition of society and suggests that

> the phenomenon of child abuse has emerged as a malign and exponential growth towards the conclusion of the 20th century not because of any significant alteration in the pattern of our behaviour towards children, but because of the changing patterns of personal, political and moral control in social life more generally which have in turn affected our vision of childhood.
>
> (ibid.: 112)

Academic discourses on the proximate causes of the current perception of an increase in child abuse are complex, and it is not appropriate to try and deal with them here. Rather we shall focus upon the broader concerns that preoccupy Jenks and upon his belief that the child becomes an important icon of any given social structure. With an heroic attempt to tidy up history, Jenks identifies the origins of the modernist child in the Enlightenment discourse of Rousseau who distils the 'principle of "care" governing the modern relationship between adults and children' and inaugurates the 'powerful commitment to childhood, in Western society, as a form of "promise"' (ibid.: 114). Thus parents give space, time and resources to their offspring, the nuclear family becomes 'the very epitome of the rational enterprise' and 'childhood is transformed into a form of human capital which, through modernity, has been dedicated to futures' (ibid.: 115). However, as the age of postmodernity approaches, the relationships that were shaped (enabled and constrained) by the nuclear family of modernity are 'outgrown'. The mastery of nature begins to imply not only control, but the possibility of self-annihilation and tradition ceases to be the platform for progress. This is the world of Beck's 'risk society' and of a reflexive self that, finding no stability for its identity in occupation, community or kin has continually to recreate itself, searching for new ways to relate to a shifting social order when '"purpose" is no longer linked to "progress"' (ibid.: 118; Beck, 1992). The impact upon childhood, argues Jenks, is profound, especially upon the way that adults perceive the state of childhood. Whilst modernism placed the child in opposition to the stability of the adult state as something changeable, fickle and in need of shaping, from within postmodernity the child appears as a fixed point, a traditional figure, an object of nostalgia. As Jenks says, 'The trust that was previously anticipated from marriage, partnership, friendship, class solidarity and so on is now invested more generally in the child' (1994: 119).

Jenks himself quotes from Beck's now classic study of 'Risk Society', but because the quotation is so redolent of the atmosphere that has surrounded much of the writing discussed in this chapter, and because it presents the 'crisis' facing childhood at its bleakest and most poignant, and most of all because it places the anguish where it belongs, not with the child but with the adult, it is worth repeating:

> The child is the source of the last remaining, irrevocable, unexchangeable primary relationship. Partners come and go. The child stays. Everything that is desired, but not realisable in the relationship, is directed to the child. With the increasing fragility of the relationship between the sexes, the child acquires a monopoly on practical companionship, on an expression of feelings in a biological give and take that otherwise is becoming increasingly uncommon and doubtful. Here an anachronistic social experience is celebrated and cultivated which has become improbable and longed for precisely because of the individualisation process. The excessive affection for children, the 'staging of childhood' which is granted to them – the poor overloved creatures – and the nasty struggle for the children during and after divorce are some symptoms of this. The child becomes the final alternative to loneliness that can be built up against the vanishing possibilities of love. It is a private type of re-enchantment, which arises with, and derives its meaning from, disenchantment.
>
> (Beck, 1992: 118)

In this context, says Jenks, to abuse a child is to attack the last icon of a disappearing social order, a jealously treasured memory of an unrecoverable past (1994: 120). Nor is it surprising that we lash out at any potential enemy of childhood; the incompetent parent or teacher, the drug-dealer, the paedophile, the maker of the video-nasty, the producer of game shows, the toy manufacturer and the television executive. Nor is it surprising that we attempt, with growing theatricality, to protect our children through fitter parenting and more accountable schools, that we visit our guilt at the impact of the

Chapter 8

The child of the millennium

Conclusion

> 'What is this doing here? This is ugly! Who is the ISBN guy? Who will buy this book anyway? Over fifty pages of nonsense and I'm only in three of them. Blah! Blah! Blah! Blah! Blah! Blah! Blah! Blah! Blah! Blah! Blah! Blah! Blah! Blah! Blah! Blah! Blah! Blah! Blah!'
>
> The Little Red Hen at the end of Scieszca and Smith's *The Stinky Cheese Man and Other Fairly Stupid Tales*

And so what of the postmodern picture book? How do we account for such a discrepancy between the joyous celebration of the playfulness of childhood, which the best of such books manifest, and the dolorous tones of those writers discussed in the previous chapter? It would of course be possible to dispute the relevance of the comparison. How, after all, can one compare a minor middle-class flourish with the depths of despair that increasingly surrounds the child in the family? Perhaps, after all, the picture book is just another consumer item (albeit one of very high quality), a way for parents to buy off their 'overloved' but uncared for children? And, perhaps, as was suggested before, even the postmodern picture book is not so innocent as it might seem. In any case, the vast majority of picture books, as Stephens has shown, are bent upon the very serious and complex business of instructing the young child about primary family relationships (Stephens, 1992). Part of the problem lies in the concept of postmodernism itself which is, as Featherstone has pointed out, an elusive idea that suffers much from its current popularity (Featherstone, 1988). Any notion that can be invoked to explain both the emergence of a certain style in picture books and the reasons for the contemporary anguish over child abuse begins to look a little shapeless.

One should not labour the point, but it is possible to be so weighed down by the concerns expressed by writers like Winn, Miles and

Postman that positive features of the state of childhood as the millennium approaches are ignored. The world of children's books still makes a small but not insignificant contribution to the life of children; the picture book has survived the coming of television and has expanded the visual literacy of many children. Print literacy will have to take its place alongside television and computer literacy, but as adults we have to take such things seriously and not simply mourn the passing of an age. It is a cliché, but one with some measure of truth in it, that it is the adult who cannot come to terms with new technologies, not the child, and the naive contrast between visual and print literacy is rapidly becoming worthless (Buckingham, 1993a). The impact of free-market economics upon the culture of children is always something that deserves the serious evaluation that Kline gives it. Nevertheless, British television at least still seeks to maintain a lively, often mature and thoughtful communication with children. Researchers like Buckingham have shown how children can take on adult television too and, collectively, make it their own (Buckingham, 1987, 1993a, b). Through television, computer technologies and old fashioned print, adults are certainly talking directly to children, and at their best (even amongst the toy manufacturers) they are seriously engaged in solving the many problems involved in representing the adult world to children through an increasing range of media.

It is, however, the erosion of the bourgeois ideology of the family that perhaps gnaws most painfully at the contemporary conscience. Women struggle to change their own circumstances whilst retaining a primary responsibility for child-rearing; men struggle to accommodate to the consequences of long-term employment insecurity in terms of both financial and social status. Both struggle to find a way of ordering their mutual relationships. The burden of history can be heavy, but even here it is possible to join Mukti Jain Campion in some brisk spring cleaning; to attempt a redefinition of parenting in terms of action rather than status, not perhaps through Total Quality Management but through something more modest that can be worked out along the way. If history does teach us anything about household and family formation, it is that it is malleable and responsive to changing circumstances. Levine has argued that the families who weathered the storm of early industrialisation did not behave as the irrational, helpless victims they are often presented as being, neither did they find their only voice through political protest. Rather, in private, they calculated the best age to get married, the best number of children to have, and how quickly to have them to maximise the chances of economic survival and perhaps even prosperity (Levine, 1987: 154f). Levine is not, of course, suggesting that people, including many children, did not suffer, but rather that in making decisions they behaved as rationally as circumstances allowed. The problems in the late twentieth century have as much to do with consciousness as economics, but ideology frequently lags behind practice precisely because the critical decisions are made by individuals according to their own private rational choices. Perhaps the most serious objection to Campion, and to any other advocate of greater state intervention in the regulation of parenting, is that no state regulation can cope with rapidly changing circumstances with the skill or knowledge of the individuals concerned, and no state offers services without ideological strings attached. One of the arguments to emerge from recent debates within developmental psychology is a challenge to the dominance of the conception of children's 'needs' as identifiable, fixed entities (Woodhead, 1990). This is normally taken to have special application to different but relatively stable practices in a cross-cultural context where 'scientific' definitions of need tend to hide their cultural origins. It also has relevance, however, to situations of rapid social change when conceptions of need can be trapped in an historic past whose relevance is fading.

DEALING WITH HISTORY

It is one thing to expect historians to write history for us, it is quite another to expect them to tell us what to do with it. Most of us, along with Foucault and with Ariès himself, are more interested in what history tells us about the present than in what it tells us about the past; more interested in looking to the past for traces of the present than in reconstructing the past for its own sake. There are some simple benefits in this, even if it is only at the level of being told that there is nothing much new in this world. And as we have seen earlier, historians themselves are not always comfortable with accounts of social change in which the state of childhood is presumed to alter too dramatically. The same kind of basic argument can be used to calm the panic of those who see contemporary childhood as being in a state of crisis. Levine, for example, offers a crumb of comfort to those who believe the family is in a state of collapse. The impact of changes in popular culture can similarly be played down. Were the old 'B' movies shown in the cinemas on Saturday mornings any better than contemporary children's television? Or are modern computer games or videos so different in their impact from some comics, or from the penny dreadfuls and chap books before them? It is always difficult to get an informed and sober judgement on such questions, but the mere raising of them makes our own situation seem less fraught. The difficulty, of course, is that on many serious issues – the nature and extent of child abuse is a clear case – history is opaque and we have no right to expect it to yield up answers; neither to make us feel better nor worse about the contemporary situation.

Lying behind this desire, however, is something more basic, to which Ariès referred when he said that he found it difficult 'to distinguish the characteristics of our living present, except by means of the differences which separate them from the related but never identical aspects of the past' (Ariès, 1973: 7). In other words, we tend always to want to evaluate our present in relation to our past, because of the simple need to establish some point of comparison, some criteria by which we can judge our current condition. And, of course, into the relationship of child to adult, there is always an in-built sense of history. Ariès offended some historians by arguing the necessity of writing history *in terms* of the present, which is a more contentious issue; but the impetus is basic to most lay approaches to history and not to be lightly dismissed on those grounds alone.

This approach is also evident in much use of history within the social sciences, where the present is the principal focus of explanation and the past is there merely to supply the chain of events that must (according to the explanation offered) lead to the present. Foucault rejected 'origins' in preference for 'beginnings' and looked for 'genealogies' rather than 'causes' in an attempt to escape the demands of the French Annales school for a causative history of the 'long period', but the temptation is always there to treat his 'beginnings' as 'origins' and his 'genealogies' as causes (Hunt, 1989). This temptation, especially within the social sciences, is always in danger of leading to a summarising of history, a collapsing of its contradictions and untidiness into a clear-cut narrative or into a set of concepts that are needed to explain the present. Thus, as we saw earlier, Ariès' study is reduced to a proposition about the 'invention' of childhood and Lawrence Stone, perhaps in a laudable desire to address a wider audience, is pushed into placing too much weight upon the concept of 'individualism' so beloved of sociological modernisation theory. Any attempt, therefore, to find traces of the past in the present should be cautious, but there is really no reason why we should not search for a narrative which will help us understand the present whilst drawing on the past. What should always be remembered, however, is that it is our reconstruction of the past, created for our purposes. We may judge ourselves by such means, but it scarcely gives us the right to judge history.

THE CHILD OF MODERNITY

The neatest story tells of the rise and fall of the bourgeois childhood. The rise was of the child as an 'object of knowledge' structured in time and space according to complex rules governing social interactions, with clearly specified norms relating to the process of growing up. This simply expressed is the thesis of Ariès and, in its basic structure, it remains the most coherent account of the emergence of the child of modernity. It also, of course, relates to Foucault's more general account of the development of discipline, examination and normalisation as technologies of power within modern society. What makes it so sturdy an account is that it is held firmly in place by a set of related discourses which appear to confirm it. Thus, it is an account of a 'bourgeois' childhood because its rise is closely associated with the story that tells of the rise of the bourgeoisie as a class. It relates to bourgeois needs in terms of cultural reproduction, their need as an emerging social as well as economic force to build up their cultural capital and to ensure generational continuity in situations where wider kinship networks were insecure. Thus childhood was identified as a separate field of human endeavour with its own internal dynamics and goals, whilst still able to mirror and anticipate the adult world. Childhood was defined above all as a learning experience, the aim of which was to position the growing child with precision in a largely preconceived individual and social space.

But the bourgeoisie as a class was one that always sensed a threat both from within, in terms of a failure of its own cultural reproduction, and from without, through the external threat of mass society. To its aid it called upon religion as a discourse offering mechanisms that provided discipline for its own children, and could also offer criteria by which to judge the behaviour of both the upper and lower classes. But religion offered more, in that, especially through Protestantism, it could structure the concept of the individual by offering conscience as a foil to conformity, principles as counters to tradition, and rationality as a spur to change. And all these qualities could become integral parts of the learning process that childhood became. Religion, too, was perhaps the discourse that allowed for an upbringing in which the gendering of socialisation produced parallel but not divergent or mutually exclusive patterns. In seeking to emphasise the differences in the upbringing of middle-class boys and girls in, for example, the Victorian period, it is possible to overlook their broad similarities. In both cases a discipline of moral restraint and the encouragement of a moral sensibility was the ideal, and in evangelical circles there was the same ultimate goal of salvation. Religion could offer a mutuality of aims across differences, underpinning a division of labour with a sense of common purpose. In sharing childhood, albeit separated by gender, the bourgeois child could learn of its place in the order of things with religion offering the vital link to a common humanity.

This is a not unfamiliar account and it is easy to see where the material in this study lends it support. In the codifying of childhood as a learning process, the tradition that stretches from the humanists through the Puritans and on to Locke (and of course others) is central. Ariès has already provided a similar far more detailed story in relation to France with particular emphasis upon the institution of the school. We may take our 'beginning' from whatever point we choose (for Ariès the Jesuits and Jansenists are critical: here, it was Locke, though it might have been Erasmus or Comenius for example), but the underlying process is the same. The child is constructed as a human being in the making, above all as a moral being in the making, whose primary duty is to learn the proper exercise of reason. Religion is never far away from this child because throughout this line of discourse religion is seen, not primarily as a means to transcendental experience, but as the discipline that guides the child upon its journey.

This study, however, has been more concerned to identify the disturbances which eddy round this general flow of ideas. In Puritanism, for example, we witnessed a certain tension between reason and fervency, possibly heightened by the impact external events had upon the dynamics of the Puritan family. There is, as Sommerville has pointed out, in the stories of Janeway a sentimentality, an emotionalism which belies the stereotypical view of Puritan repressiveness; and Leverenz has pointed to the tension that existed for parents in the contrasting roles of tender mother and grave governor (Sommerville, 1982; Leverenz, 1980). Because the label Puritan has been so much abused for the last 400 years or so, it is difficult now to capture the range of possibilities that lay within its perception of childhood. No doubt there were repressive Puritans, but they lived alongside rational

Puritans and highly emotional Puritans, and probably also alongside many who genuinely tried to achieve the balance between love and discipline, between reason and feeling that was their ideal.

Possibly the evangelicals of the late eighteenth and early nineteenth centuries kept their emotions more firmly under control, but as their influence spread, they were assaulted by new sources of disturbance. In Rousseau, as we have seen, there was an ambiguous legacy and in Romanticism itself there were conceptions of childhood subversive of the whole religious, rationalist project. It is sometimes suggested that the innocent child of Romanticism somehow replaced the older view of the child as the inheritor of original sin, but this was never the case. Rather the two conceptions whirled around each other, producing as Grylls says 'weird patterns of thought', but also producing that brilliant, sometimes enchanting, occasionally infuriating gallery of images that presents nineteenth-century society to us in all its contradictions – Francis Wayland and Letitia Landon, Mr Barlow and Charles Dickens, Henty's heroes and Little Lord Fauntleroy, Daisy Ashford and *The Little Mermaid* (Grylls, 1978). It would be wrong, however, to suggest that Romanticism did not leave its mark. It is, along with Rousseau, one of many 'beginnings' of discourses which feed into the twentieth-century's idea of childhood. What, for example, has been relatively little explored is the way in which discourses coming from science construct the innocence of the child. Brief mention has been made of recapitulation theories as echoes of Romantic naturalism, but there is in developmentalism generally a certain desire to protect the child from a too invasive, too rational adult presence. There are, of course, competing scientific discourses coming from behaviourism and from the hygienists, to say nothing of psychoanalysis, but these are beyond the scope of this study (Beekman, 1978; Hardyment, 1984; Dwork, 1987). What remains indisputable is that the notion of childhood innocence with all the cultural weight that it brings with it from the nineteenth century and beyond is a belief that has come to haunt us and often mock us in the late twentieth century. Less and less do we believe that we can sustain the conditions in which childhood innocence is possible.

Another source of disturbance for the discourse upon the bourgeois child was sex. As far as we know, it was only at the extreme edge of the Puritan sects that sexuality became an issue, but for the Victorians the whole issue became more problematic. The problem, as Kincaid insists, lies in the way we construct the child as innocent and then find that very innocence erotic (Kincaid, 1992). Childhood sexuality is antithetical to the bourgeois conception not only because it allows the child to escape from its pre-ordained childhood schedule, but also because it connects the child to the adult in ways which destroy the sense of adult distance and control. Just as the female was always potentially dangerous to the Victorian male equilibrium, so was the beauty of the child. In the hands of Lewis Carroll, perhaps (though Carol Mavor is not entirely sure), the child found a unique voice, a unique chance to reply, to gaze back at the photographer and to take possession of the photograph (Mavor, 1994). But Victorian society could not accept; Carroll stopped taking photographs and the imagination which produced *Alice* dwindled away to dream of fairies. In bourgeois discourse, marriage is the appointed time for sex, and childhood is merely a preparation for it, a time of gathering reason. But Rousseau knew that passion would come before then whether or not we wished it, and Romanticism knew that in childhood is a beauty so breathtaking that adults cannot but long to take possession.

The story of the rise of the bourgeois child is now also the story of the fall of the bourgeois child. Here, Ariès' explanation (now well over thirty years old) looks distinctly old-fashioned. His concern was for the introverted nature of the modern nuclear family, lavishing 'obsessive love' upon the child, intolerant of variety (Ariès, 1973: 398). What hope now for that vanishing institution, the nuclear family? It is easy to see why, in our narrative, the fall must come. The class structure that sustained the bourgeois child is fragmenting; popular culture, the media and the marketers leave 'standards' in tatters, breaking the rules and tearing down the boundaries which defended the place of bourgeois culture; gone are the rules of cultural transmission by which the child reached this place of safety. Discipline has gone with religion since there is in secular society no force beyond the self, no reference point beyond mere intersubjectivities, only a fragile, precarious understanding of a possible shared meaning.

This was the message conveyed so passionately by the writers discussed in the previous chapter. The discourse cannot hold. The sentimentality that lurked alongside Puritan fervency and that crippled Romanticism's attempt to represent the child of nature now holds full sway as the sentimentalised child lisps its cute way through the realms of popular culture. The designer child has its brief hour of glory but is then discarded and the child as victim gazes down at us from the charity posters, wide-eyed and hungry, demanding that our love, our money and our anger be expended on its behalf. The sexualised child and the asexual child tumble over each other in their desire to command our attention. In teenage magazines young teenage girls learn how to cope with 'boyf's' more urgent demands, and dancing at the school show in front of parents and teachers, they practise their pelvic thrusts with more ignorance than innocence. At the same time, they are taught to fear the streets at night, to spurn the smile of the stranger and to evade the embrace of an uncle. Meanwhile adult rationality runs wild as the state, educators and health lobbyists compete over how, where and when children should be introduced to the adult world of sexuality, pursuing the bourgeois child with standards and with reasons, when that child has long since heard other voices, slipped under their arm and gone its own way.

It is as if those disturbances that threatened the story of the bourgeois child had finally come into their own and overwhelmed it, not just offering minor digressions along the way or adding spice to a plain tale, but reshaping and rewriting the narrative completely. But there is a danger in extrapolating from these tales of woe to the actual experience of children, not least because to do so is often to ignore the spontaneous responses of those most involved, both parents and children. Late twentieth-century children are probably no more dominated by television than their Victorian ancestors were dominated by their parents, or their Puritan ancestors by religion. Puritan children believed in the real possibility of salvation and in the real possibility of hell, and some no doubt became obsessed, but most played and learned and eventually got on with the business of finding a partner and earning a living. Bourgeois Victorian children believed in the separate roles allotted to them, boy and girl, and in the rightness of the adult duties they were learning to perform. Some, no doubt, lived in a state of resentful dependence upon their parents (and perhaps some even upon their school), but most had to learn how to negotiate parental ideals against a reality in which survival and defence of status were paramount. Late twentieth-century children perhaps have more negotiation to do from an earlier age, more competing sources of knowledge to handle, less certainty in the futures adults project before them. As 'objects of knowledge', they are less easily constructed in discourse, but there are freedoms and possibilities in this. Ariès himself might have welcomed this return to his vision of the heyday of childhood in the *ancien régime*, a time of 'gay indifference' on the part of fathers when the 'old sociabilities' offered far greater scope for individualism, before schools and the bourgeois family achieved their control (Ariès, 1973: 393).

It is actually a very foolish kind of cost–benefit analysis that tries to evaluate one period as being better for children than any other; there are too many variables and no absolute criteria with which to make comparisons. What we can do is to identify and contemplate in our various roles as parents, teachers, child-professionals, 'experts' and so on, the problems and possibilities that lie in any particular direction contemporary discourse might take. There is much that writers such as Winn, Miles, Postman and Kline say which should be taken seriously, but there are perhaps two more general issues which are worth identifying as contemporary features of discourse. Both have serious implications for the way in which we interact with children, devise policies that influence their lives and develop institutions in conjunction with which they have to live.

The first has to do with the role of 'modesty' in the relations between benefactor and beneficiary, identified by Judith Still as an important, if somewhat hidden preoccupation of Rousseau. If there is an immanent tendency in discourses relating to the child of modernity which shows no sign of lessening in the late twentieth century it is the demand for ever greater disclosure of the child to the adult. The child of late twentieth-century discourse is left with little modesty, little with which to protect itself from the invasions of the adult. This is the child of Bernstein's invisible pedagogy, deprived of knowing the rules of the game itself, but encouraged through play to 'exteriorise' itself to adult surveillance (Bernstein, 1977: 121). This is Postman's child, for whom nothing is shameful; who, because adults have no secrets, can have none of its own. There are more radical discourses which attempt to deal with this, most obviously by extrapolating from a fundamentally liberal discourse to talk of children's rights, but these are too easily swallowed up by adult advocacy on behalf of children. And then perhaps the greatest danger, as Kincaid suggests, lies in our response to the problem we have ourselves created; the danger of beginning to see all relations with children as relations of power (Kincaid, 1992: 16f). As in some feminisms when all sexual relations between men and women are seen as rape because of the unequal relations existing between men and women, so between adult and child all relations come to be seen as unequal relations from which the child must be defended. And in despair, in an attempt to protect, we demand even greater disclosure of the child to the adult. Children may play – we will protect their right to do so – but no longer may we play with them lest we miss some significance, some meaning in what they do.

The second tendency from which there seems little escape is that which connects the child to the adult through autobiography. At the end of the seventeenth century, Pierre Bayle seemed to suggest that the only way for the human race to escape its inherently tragic fate was for the adult to reject its own childhood. In denying that possibility, Locke, Wordsworth and so many others who have shaped modern childhood have not only contributed to the denial of the commonality of much human experience, but have denied to many an escape route from unhappiness, the chance to reject what they once were. It is, as Easthope suggests (in reference to Wordsworth's most famous line, 'I wandered lonely as a cloud'), a special kind of loneliness that derives from the narcissism inherent in the search for the self (Easthope, 1993: 127). Indifference to childhood, gay or otherwise, is no longer possible but it is possible to demand too much of children, especially by failing to acknowledge that the adult role of benefactor should be shaped by the need for modesty in all transactions with children. It is also possible to demand too much from our own childhoods. We need to distinguish between the need that Dickens recognised for a certain childishness to remain with us as adults, and the desire to cling on to our own individual history. What is important is not the memory, which in any case is almost certainly illusory, but the possibility of finding in childish things, and with luck in children themselves, a renewed humanity. The great contribution Wordsworth made was to see in the child the possibility of renewed hope and life; his more problematic legacy was to see in that child, himself. It is responsibility enough to create images of childhood and visit them upon the next generation, without trying to make ourselves in the image of our own past childhood.

References

Pre-twentieth century stories and poems for children have not been formally referenced here. With the exception of a few very famous stories from later in the century, which are available in a bewildering variety of editions, they are mostly now out of print and copies are not readily accessible, though they can be found in specialist libraries and collections. References to specific editions would not therefore serve much practical purpose. But for those who wish to learn more there could be no better place to start than with Brian Alderson's revision of F. J. Harvey Darton's *Children's Books in England*, or Peter Hunt's *International Companion Encyclopedia of Children's Literature*, and for those who wish themselves to read these stories and poems a good place to start would be with Tessa Rose Chester's *Children's Books Research: A Practical Guide to Techniques and Sources*

Adrian, A.A. (1984) *Dickens and the Parent–Child Relationship*, Athens: Ohio University Press.

Ahlberg, J. and A. (1985) *The Jolly Postman or Other People's Letters*, London: Heineman.

Andrews, M. (1994) *Dickens and the Grown-up Child*, Basingstoke: Macmillan.

Archard, D. (1993) *Children: Rights and Childhood*, London: Routledge.

Ariès, P. (1973) *Centuries of Childhood*, Harmondsworth: Penguin.

Armitage, D.M. (1939) *The Taylors of Ongar*, Cambridge: W. Heffer & Sons.

Ashfield, A. (ed.) (1995) *Romantic Women Poets, 1770–1838: An Anthology*, Manchester: Manchester University Press.

Ashford, D. (1919) *The Young Visiters*, London: Chatto & Windus.

—— (1983) *The Hangman's Daughter and Other Stories*, Oxford: Oxford University Press.

Auerbach, N. (1982) *Woman and the Demon: The Life of a Victorian Myth*, Cambridge, Mass.: Harvard University Press.

—— (1986) *Romantic Imprisonment: Women and Other Glorified Outcasts*, New York: Columbia University Press.

Badinter, E. (1981) *The Myth of Motherhood: An Historical View of the Maternal Instinct*, trans. Roger DeGaris, London: Souvenir Press.

Bantock, G.H. (1980) *Studies in the History of Educational Theory: Volume 1, Artifice and Nature, 1350–1765*, London: George Allen & Unwin.
Barry, K. (1979) *Female Sexual Slavery*, New York: New York University Press.
Barthes, R. (1973) *Mythologies*, trans. Annette Lavers, London: Palladin, HarperCollins.
Batchelor, J. (1989) 'Dodgson, Carroll, and the emancipation of Alice' in Avery, G. and Briggs J. (eds) *Children and their Books: A Celebration of the Work of Iona and Peter Opie*, Oxford: Clarendon Press.
Baumer, F.L. (1977) *Modern European Thought: Continuity and Change in Ideas, 1600–1950*, New York: Macmillan.
BBC (1994) 'The End of Childhood?', *Late Show*, BBC2, 5 December.
Beck, U. (1992) *Risk Society: Towards a New Modernity*, trans. Mark Ritter, London: Sage.
Beekman, D. (1978) *The Mechanical Baby: A Popular History of the Theory and Practice of Child Raising*, New York: Meridian.
Berger, B. and P. (1983) *The War Over the Family: Capturing the Middle Ground*, London: Hutchinson.
Bernstein, B. (1977) *Class, Codes and Control*, Vol. 3, 2nd edn, London: Routledge & Kegan Paul.
Best, J. (ed.) (1994) *Troubling Children: Studies of Children and Social Problems*, New York: Aldine de Gruyter.
Blumler, J.G. (1992) *The Future of Children's Television in Britain: An Enquiry for the Broadcasting Standards Council*, London: Broadcasting Standards Council.
Brannen, J. and O'Brien, M. (eds) (1995a) *Childhood and Parenthood*, London: Institute of Education, University of London.
—— (1995b) 'Childhood and the sociological gaze: paradigms and paradoxes', *Sociology*, 29(4): 729–37.
Bratton, J.S. (1981) *The Impact of Victorian Children's Fiction*, London: Croom Helm.
Breen, J. (ed.) (1992) *Women Romantic Poets, 1785–1832: An Anthology*, London: Dent.
Bremer, F.J. (1976) *The Puritan Experiment*, New York: St Martin's Press.
Briggs, J. (1995) 'Transitions (1890–1914)' in Hunt, P. (ed.) (1995) *Children's Literature: An Illustrated History*, Oxford: Oxford University Press.
Briggs, J. and Butts, D. (1995) 'The emergence of form (1850–1890)' in Hunt, P. (ed.) (1995) *Children's Literature: An Illustrated History*, Oxford: Oxford University Press.
Broome, J.H. (1963) *Rousseau*, London: Arnold.
Brown, M. (1993) 'Romanticism and the Enlightenment' in Curren, S. (ed.) *The Cambridge Companion to British Romanticism*, Cambridge: Cambridge University Press.
Browne, A. (1982) *Bear Goes to Town*, London: Arrow Books, Hutchinson.
—— (1995) *Through the Magic Mirror*, Harmondsworth: Picture Puffin.
Buckingham, D. (1987) *Public Secrets: Eastenders and Its Audience*, London: British Film Institute.
—— (1993a) *Children Talking Television: The Making of Television Literacy*, London: The Falmer Press.

—— (ed.) (1993b) *Reading Audiences: Young People and the Media*, Manchester: Manchester University Press.

Burningham, J. (1984) *Grandpa*, London: Jonathan Cape.

—— (1992) *Come away from the water, Shirley*, London: Random House.

Burstyn, J. (1980) *Victorian Education and the Ideal of Womanhood*, London: Croom Helm.

Butts, D. (1995) 'The beginnings of Victorianism (c1820–1850)' in Hunt, P. (ed.) (1995) *Children's Literature: An Illustrated History*, Oxford: Oxford University Press.

Campion, M.J. (1995) *Who's Fit to Be a Parent?*, London: Routledge.

Carpenter, H. (1985) *Secret Gardens: A Study of the Golden Age of Children's Literature*, London: George Allen & Unwin.

Casey, J. (1989) *The History of the Family*, Oxford: Blackwell.

Charvet, J. (1974) *The Social Problem in the Philosophy of Rousseau*, Cambridge: Cambridge University Press.

Chester, T.R. (1989) *Children's Books Research: A Practical Guide to Techniques and Sources*, Stroud: Thimble Press.

Cohen, M.N. (1984) 'Lewis Carroll and Victorian morality' in Don Richard Cox (ed.) *Sexuality and Victorian Literature*, Tennessee: Tennessee University Press.

Cole, E.W. and Hope, E. (eds) (n.d.) *The Thousand Best Poems in the World*, London: Hutchinson & Co.

Coveney, P. (1967) *The Image of Childhood*, Harmondsworth: Penguin.

Crocker, L.G. (1973) *Jean-Jacques Rousseau*, New York: Macmillan.

Cunningham, H. (1991) *The Children of the Poor: Representations of Childhood Since the Seventeenth Century*, Oxford: Blackwell.

Darton, J. Harvey (1982)[1932] *Children's Books in England*, 3rd edn, revised by Brian Alderson, Cambridge: Cambridge University Press.

Davidoff, L. (1979) 'Class and gender in Victorian England: the diaries of Arthur J. Munby and Hannah Cullwick', *Feminist Studies*, 5(1): 87–141.

Davidoff, L. and Hall, C. (1987) *Family Fortunes: Men and Women of the English Middle Class, 1780–1850*, London: Hutchinson.

De Morgan (1886) Letter in *The Athenaeum*, No. 2011.

Demos, J. (1970) *A Little Commonwealth: Family Life in Plymouth Colony*, New York: Oxford University Press.

Dillon, G.M. (1976) 'Policy and dramaturgy: a critique of current conceptions of policy making', *Policy and Politics*, 5: 47–62.

Donzelot, J. (1980) *The Policing of Families*, trans. Robert Hurley, London: Hutchinson.

Doran, S. and Durston, C. (1991) *Princes, Pastors and People: The Church and Religion in England, 1529–1689*, London: Routledge.

Dunn, J. (1984) *Locke*, Oxford: Oxford University Press.

Durston, C. (1989) *The Family in the English Revolution*, Oxford: Blackwell.

Dwork, D. (1987) *War is Good for Babies and Other Young Children: A History of the Infant and Child Welfare Movement in England*, 1898–1918, New York: Tavistock Publications.

Dyhouse, C. (1981) *Girls Growing Up in Late Victorian and Edwardian England*, London: Routledge & Kegan Paul.

Eagleton, T. (1983) *Literary Theory: An Introduction*, Oxford: Blackwell.

Easthope, A. (1993) *Wordsworth Now and Then: Romanticism and Contemporary Culture*, Buckingham: Open University Press.
Elkind, D. (1981) *The Hurried Child: Growing Up Too Fast Too Soon*, Reading, Mass.: Addison-Wesley.
Empson, W. (1935) *Some Versions of Pastoral*, London: Chatto & Windus.
Fairchild, H.N. (1961) [1928] *The Noble Savage: A Study in Romantic Naturalism*, New York: Russell & Russell.
Fairclough, N. (1992) *Discourse and Social Change*, Cambridge: Polity.
Featherstone, M. (1988) 'In pursuit of the postmodern: an introduction', *Theory, Culture and Society*, 5(2–3): 195–215.
Foucault, M. (1984) *The History of Sexuality, Volume 1: An Introduction*, trans. Robert Hurley, Harmondsworth: Penguin.
Garden, M. (1970) *Lyon et les Lyonnais au XVIIIe Siècle*, Paris: Les Belles Lettres.
Gaull, M. (1988) *English Romanticism: The Human Context*, New York: W.W. Norton.
Gillis, J. (1979) 'Affective individualism and the English poor', *Journal of Interdisciplinary History*, 10, Summer: 121–8.
Gorham, D. (1978) 'The "Maiden Tribute of Modern Babylon" re-examined: child prostitution and the idea of childhood in late Victorian England', *Victorian Studies*, 21(3): 353–79.
—— (1982) *The Victorian Girl and the Feminine Ideal*, London: Croom Helm.
Greven, P. (1977) *The Protestant Temperament: Patterns of Child-Rearing, Religious Experience, and the Self in Early America*, New York: Knopf.
Grey, D.J. (ed.) (1992) *Lewis Carroll, Alice In Wonderland: Backgrounds, Essays in Criticism*, 2nd edn, New York: W.W. Norton.
Grylls, D. (1978) *Guardians and Angels: Parents and Children in Nineteenth Century Literature*, London: Faber & Faber.
Guiliano, E. (ed.) (1982) *Lewis Carroll: A Celebration: Essays on the Occasion of the 150th Anniversary of the Birth of Charles Lutwidge Dodgson*, New York: Clarkson N. Potter.
Gunter, B. and McAleer, J.L. (1990) *Children and Television: The One Eyed Monster*, London: Routledge.
Hampson, N. (1968) *The Enlightenment*, Harmondsworth: Penguin.
Hardyment, C. (1984) *Dream Babies: Child Care from Locke to Spock*, Oxford: Oxford University Press.
Hendrick, H. (1990) 'Constructions and reconstructions of British childhood: an interpretive survey, 1800 to the present' in James, A. and Prout, A. (eds) *Constructing and Reconstructing Childhood: Contemporary Issues in the Sociological Study of Childhood*, Basingstoke: Falmer Press.
Heywood, J. (1965) *Children in Care: The Development of the Service for the Deprived Child*, 2nd edn, London: Routledge & Kegan Paul.
Hill, C. (1964) *Society and Puritanism in Pre-Revolutionary England*, London: Secker & Warburg.
—— (1980) *The Century of Revolution: 1603–1714*, 2nd edn, Walton-on-Thames: Nelson.
Hodge, R. and Kress, G. (1988) *Social Semiotics*, Cambridge: Polity.
Hodge, R and Tripp, D. (1986) *Children and Television: A Semiotic Approach*, Cambridge: Polity.

Holme, B. (1976) *The Kate Greenaway Book*, New York: The Viking Press.

Houlbrooke, R. (1984) *The English Family: 1450–1700*, London: Longman.

Hunt, D. (1972) *Parents and Children: the Psychology of Family Life in Early Modern France*, New York: Harper & Row.

Hunt, L. (1986) 'French history in the last twenty years: the rise and fall of the *Annales* paradigm', *Journal of Contemporary History*, 21: 209–24.

—— (ed.) (1989) *The New Cultural History*, California: University of California Press.

Hunt, P. (1991) *Criticism, Theory and Children's Literature*, Oxford: Blackwell.

—— (ed.) (1992) *Literature for Children: Contemporary Criticism*, London: Routledge.

—— (1994) *An Introduction to Children's Literature*, Oxford: Oxford University Press.

—— (ed.) (1995) *Children's Literature: An Illustrated History*, Oxford: Oxford University Press.

—— (1996) *International Companion Encyclopedia of Children's Literature*, London: Routledge.

Hutton, P.H. (1981) 'The history of mentalités: the new map of cultural history', *History and Theory*, 20(3): 237–59.

James, A. and Jenks, C. (1994) 'Public perceptions of childhood criminality', unpublished paper given at ESRC seminar, University of Keele.

James, A. and Prout, A. (eds) (1990) *Constructing and Reconstructing Childhood: Contemporary Issues in the Sociological Study of Childhood*, London: Falmer Press.

Jeffreys, S. (1985) *The Spinster and her Enemies: Feminism and Sexuality, 1880–1930*, London: Pandora.

Jenks, C. (ed.) (1982) *The Sociology of Childhood: Essential Readings*, London: Batsford.

—— (1994) 'Child abuse in the postmodern context: an issue of identity' *Childhood*, 2: 111–21.

Kessen, W. (ed.) (1965) *The Child*, New York: Wiley.

Kincaid, J.R. (1973) 'Alice's invasion of Wonderland', *PMLA*, 88(1): 92–9.

—— (1992) *Child-Loving: The Erotic Child and Victorian Culture*, New York: Routledge.

Kline, S. (1993) *Out of the Garden: Toys, TV and Children's Culture in the Age of Marketing*, London and New York: Verso.

Labrousse, E. (1964) *Pierre Bayle*, Vol. 2, The Hague: Nijhof.

—— (1983) *Bayle*, Oxford: Oxford University Press.

La Bruyère, J. (1963) *Characters*, trans. H. van Lann, Oxford: Oxford University Press.

Lang, L.B. (1976) [1893] 'The Fairchild family and their creator' in Salway, L. (ed.) *A Peculiar Gift: Nineteenth Century Writing on Books for Children*, Harmondsworth: Kestrel Books.

Leites, E. (1981) 'Locke's liberal theory of parenthood' in Brandt, R. (ed.) *John Locke: Symposium Wolfenbuttel*, Berlin: Walter de Gruyter.

Leverenz, D. (1980) *The Language of Puritan Feeling: An Exploration in Literature, Psychology, and Social History*, New Jersey: Rutgers University Press.

Levine, D. (1987) *Reproducing Families: The Political Economy of English Population History*, Cambridge: Cambridge University Press.

Lewis, D. (1990) 'The constructedness of texts: picture books and the metafictive' *Signal*, 62: 131–46.

Lloyd, G. (1984) *The Man of Reason: 'Male' and 'Female' in Western Philosophy*, London: Methuen.

Locke, J. (1978) [1690] *Two Treatises of Government*, Everyman Edition, London: Dent.

—— (1989) [1693] *Some Thoughts Concerning Education*, edited by Yolton, J.W. and J.S., New York: Oxford University Press.

Lonsdale, R. (ed.) (1989) *Eighteenth Century Women Poets: An Oxford Anthology*, Oxford: Oxford University Press.

Lovejoy, A.O. (1936) *The Great Chain of Being: A Study of the History of an Idea*, Cambridge, Mass.: Harvard University Press.

Macfarlane, A. (1970) *The Family Life of Ralph Josselin*, Cambridge: Cambridge University Press.

—— (ed.) (1976) *The Diary of Ralph Josselin*, Oxford: Oxford University Press.

—— (1979) Review of Stone, L. (1977), *History and Theory*, 18: 103–125.

McKendrick, N. (1974) 'Home demand and economic growth: a new view of the role of women and children in the industrial revolution' in McKendrick, N. (ed.) *Historical Perspectives: Studies in English Thought and Society*, London: Europa.

Mackenzie, D. (ed.) (1993) Introduction to Rudyard Kipling, *Puck of Pook's Hill* and *Rewards and Fairies*, Oxford: Oxford University Press.

McLoughlin, W.G. (1975) 'Evangelical childrearing in the age of Jackson: Francis Wayland's view on when and how to subdue the wilfulness of children', *Journal of Social History*, 9, Fall: 20–43.

Mangan, J.A. and Walvin, J. (eds) (1987) *Manliness and Morality: Middle Class Masculinity in Britain and America, 1800–1940*, Manchester: Manchester University Press.

Manheimer, J. (1979) 'Murderous mothers: the problem of parenting in the Victorian novel', *Feminist Studies*, 5(3): 530–46.

Marcus, S. (1967) *The Other Victorians: A Study of Sexuality and Pornography in Mid Nineteenth Century England*, London: Weidenfeld & Nicolson.

Mason, M. (1994a) *The Making of Victorian Sexuality*, Oxford: Oxford University Press.

—— (1994b) *The Making of Victorian Sexual Attitudes*, Oxford: Oxford University Press.

Masters, R.D. (1968) *The Political Philosophy of Rousseau*, Princeton: Princeton University Press.

Mause, Ll. de (ed.) (1976) *The History of Childhood: The Evolution of Parent–Child Relationships as a Factor in History*, London: Souvenir Press.

Mavor, C. (1994) 'Dream-rushes: Lewis Carroll's photographs of the little girl' in Nelson, C. and Vallone, L. (eds) *The Girl's Own: Cultural Histories of the Anglo-American Girl, 1830–1915*, Athens: University of Georgia Press.

May, M. (1973) 'Innocence and experience: the evolution of the concept of juvenile delinquency in the mid-nineteenth century', *Victorian Studies*, 17: 7–29.

Mayall, B. (ed.) (1994) *Children's Childhoods: Observed and Experienced*, London: Falmer Press.

Mellor, A.K. (1993) *Romanticism and Gender*, New York: Routledge.

Meyrowitz, J. (1984) 'The adultlike child and the childlike adult: socialisation in an electronic age', *Daedalus*, Summer: 19–48.

Midgely, G. (ed.) (1980) *The Poems of John Bunyan*, Oxford: Clarendon Press.

Miles, R. (1994) *The Children We Deserve: Love and Hate in the Making of the Family*, London: HarperCollins.

Millett, K. (1972) 'The debate over women: Ruskin vs. Mill' in Vicinus, M. (ed.) *Suffer and Be Still: Women in the Victorian Age*, Bloomington: Indiana University Press.

Morgan, E.S. (1958) *The Puritan Dilemma: The Story of John Winthrop*, Boston: Little, Brown and Co.

—— (1966) *The Puritan Family: Religion and Domestic Relations in Seventeenth-Century New England*, New York: Harper & Row.

Morgan, J. (1986) *Godly Learning: Puritan Attitudes towards Reason, Learning, and Education*, Cambridge: Cambridge University Press.

Morton, A.L. (1978) 'Pilgrim's Progress', *History Workshop Journal*, 5, Spring.

Moss, G. (1992) 'Metafiction, illustration, and the poetics of children's literature' in Hunt, P. (ed.) *Literature for Children: Contemporary Criticism*, London: Routledge.

Neill, A. (1991) 'Locke on habituation, autonomy and education' in Ashcraft, R. (ed.) *John Locke: Critical Assessments*, Vol. 2, London: Routledge.

Nelson, C. (1989) 'Sex and the single boy: ideals of manliness and sexuality in Victorian literature for boys', *Victorian Studies*, Summer: 525–50.

Neuman, R.P. (1974) 'Masturbation, madness, and the modern concepts of childhood and adolescence', *Journal of Social History*, 8: 1–27.

O'Brien, P. (1989) 'Michel Foucault's history of culture' in Hunt, L. (ed.) *The New Cultural History*, California: University of California Press.

O'Day, R. (1982) *Education and Society, 1500–1800: The Social Foundations of Education in Early Modern Britain*, London: Longman.

Okin, S.M. (1980) *Women in Western Political Thought*, London: Virago.

Opie, I. (1993) *The People in the Playground*, Oxford: Oxford University Press.

Opie, I. and P. (1959) *The Lore and Language of Schoolchildren*, Oxford: Oxford University Press.

—— (1969) *Children's games in Street and Playground*, Oxford: Oxford University Press.

—— (1985) *The Singing Game*, Oxford: Oxford University Press.

O'Sullivan, T., Hartley, J., Saunders, D., Montgomery, M., and Fiske, J. (1994 2nd edn) *Key Concepts in Communication and Cultural Studies*, 2nd edn, London: Routledge.

Parry, G. (1978) *John Locke*, London: George Allen & Unwin.

Passmore, J. (1970) *The Perfectibility of Man*, London: Duckworth.

Pattison, R. (1978) *The Child Figure in English Literature*, Athens: University of Georgia Press.

Pearsall, R. (1983) *The Worm in the Bud: The World of Victorian Sexuality*, Harmondsworth: Penguin.
Petrie, G. (1971) *A Singular Iniquity: The Campaigns of Josephine Butler*, London: Macmillan.
Phillips, R. (ed.) (1972) *Aspects of Alice: Lewis Carroll's Dreamchild As Seen Through the Critic's Looking-Glasses*, Harmondsworth: Penguin.
Pinchbeck, I. and Hewitt, M. (1973) *Children in English Society*, Vol. 2, London: Routledge & Kegan Paul.
Pinney, T. (ed.) (1963) *Essays of George Eliot*, London: Routledge & Kegan Paul.
Plowden, A. (1974) *The Case of Eliza Armstrong: 'A Child of 13 Bought for £5'*, London: British Broadcasting Corporation.
Plumb, J.H. (1975) 'The new world of childhood in eighteenth century England', *Past and Present*, 67: 64–95.
Pollock, L. (1983) *Forgotten Children: Parent–Child Relations from 1500 to 1900*, Cambridge: Cambridge University Press.
—— (1987) *A Lasting Relationship: Parents and Children Over Three Centuries*, London: Fourth Estate.
Porter, R. (1990) *The Enlightenment*, Basingstoke: Macmillan.
Postman, N. (1983) *The Disappearance of Childhood*, London: W.H. Allen.
Quigly, I. (1987) Introduction to Rudyard Kipling, *The Complete Stalky & Co.*,Oxford: Oxford University Press.
Qvortrup, J. (1990) 'A voice for children in statistical and social accounting: a plea for children's right to be heard' in James, A. and Prout, A. (eds) *Constructing and Reconstructing Childhood: Contemporary Issues in the Sociological Study of Childhood*, Basingstoke: Falmer Press.
—— (1991) *Childhood as a Social Phenomenon – An Introduction to a Series of National Reports*, 2nd edn, Vienna: European Centre for Social Welfare Policy and Research.
—— (1994) *Childhood Matters: Social Theory, Practice and Politics*, Aldershot: Avebury.
Richards, J. (1982) 'Spreading the gospel of self-help: G.A. Henty and Samuel Smiles', *The Journal of Popular Culture*, 16(2): 52–65.
—— (1988) *Happiest Days: The Public Schools in English Fiction*, Manchester: Manchester University Press.
Roberts, H.E. (1972) 'Marriage, redundancy and sin: the painter's view of women in the first twenty-five years of Victoria's reign' in Vicinus, M. (ed.) *Suffer and Be Still: Women in the Victorian Age*, Bloomington: Indiana University Press.
Rousseau, J.-J. (1973) [1762, 1750, 1754] *The Social Contract and Discourses*, trans. G.D.H. Cole, Everyman Edition, London: Dent.
—— (1979) [1762] *Emile or On Education*, trans. Allan Bloom, New York: Basic Books.
Rusk, R. (1979, 5th ed. revised Scotland, J.) *The Doctrines of the Great Educators*, 5th edn, London: Macmillan.
Salway, L. (ed.) (1976) *A Peculiar Gift: Nineteenth Century Writings on Books for Children*, Harmondsworth: Kestrel Books.
Sarup, M. (1992) *Jaques Lacan*, New York: Harvester Wheatsheaf.

Sasek, L.A. (1989) *Images of English Puritanism: A Collection of Documentary Sources, 1589–1646*, Baton Rouge: Louisiana State University Press.

Schochet, G.J. (1975) *Patriarchalism and Political Thought*, Oxford: Blackwell.

Schouls, P.A. (1992) *Reasoned Freedom: John Locke and Enlightenment*, Ithaca: Cornell University Press.

Schucking, L.L. (1969) *The Puritan Family: a Social Study from the Literary Sources*, trans. Brian Battershaw, London: Routledge & Kegan Paul.

Schultz, R.L. (1972) *Crusader in Babylon: W.T. Stead and the Pall Mall Gazette*, Lincoln: University of Nebraska Press.

Scieszka, J. and Smith, L. (1991) *The True Story of the 3 Little Pigs by A. Wolf*, Harmondsworth: Picture Puffin.

—— (1993) *The Stinky Cheese Man and Other Fairly Stupid Tales*, Harmondsworth: Picture Puffin.

Sendak, M. (1970) *Where The Wild Things Are*, Harmondsworth: Picture Puffin.

—— (1973) *In the Night Kitchen*, Harmondsworth: Picture Puffin.

Sheridan, A. (1980) *Michel Foucault: The Will to Truth*, London: Tavistock.

Smith, F.B. (1979) *The People's Health: 1830–1910*, London: Croom Helm.

Sommerville, C.J. (1982) *The Rise and Fall of Childhood*, Beverly Hills: Sage.

—— (1992) *The Discovery of Childhood in Puritan England*, Athens, USA: University of Georgia Press.

Spellman, W.M. (1988) *John Locke and the Problem of Depravity*, Oxford: Clarendon Press.

Spilka, M. (1984) 'On the enrichment of poor monkeys by myth and dream; or, how Dickens Rousseauisticized and pre-Freudianised Victorian views of childhood' in Don Richard Cox (ed.) *Sexuality and Victorian Literature*, Tennessee: Tennessee University Press.

Stainton Rogers, R. and W. (1992) *Stories of Childhood: Shifting Agendas of Child Concern*, Hemel Hempstead: Harvester Wheatsheaf.

Stannard, D.E. (1977) *The Puritan Way of Death: A Study of Religion, Culture and Social Change*, New York: Oxford University Press.

Stephens, J. (1992) *Language, Ideology and Children's Fiction*, Harlow: Longman.

Stewart, C.D. (1975) *The Taylors of Ongar* (2 volumes), London: Garland Publishing.

Still, J. (1993) *Justice and Difference in the Works of Rousseau*, Cambridge: Cambridge University Press.

Stocker, M. (1992) 'From faith to reason? Religious thought in the seventeenth century' in Cain, T.G.S. and Robinson, K. (eds) *Into Another Mould: Change and Continuity in English Culture, 1625–1700*, London: Routledge.

Stone, L. (1975) 'The rise of the nuclear family in early modern England' in Rosenberg, C.E. (ed.) *The Family in History*, Philadelphia: University of Pennsylvania Press.

—— (1977) *The Family, Sex and Marriage in England: 1500–1800*, London: Weidenfeld & Nicolson.

—— (1979) *The Family, Sex and Marriage in England: 1500–1800*, abridged edn, Harmondsworth: Penguin.

Thompson, E.P. (1977) 'Happy families', *New Society*, 8 September: 499–501.

Todd, M. (1980) 'Humanists, Puritans and the spiritualised household', *Church History*, 49: 18–34.

—— (1987) *Christian Humanism and the Puritan Social Order*, Cambridge: Cambridge University Press.

Tomalin, C. (ed.) (1981) *Parents and Children*, Oxford: Oxford University Press.

Trumbach, R. (1978) *The Rise of the Egalitarian Family*, New York: Academic Press.

Unstead, R.J. (1955) *Looking at History*, London: A. & C. Black.

Van Evra, J. (1990) *Television and Child Development*, New Jersey: Lawrence Erlbaum Associates.

Vann, R.T. (1982) 'The youth of *Centuries of Childhood*', *History and Theory*, 21(2): 279–97.

Vicinus, M. (ed.) (1972) *Suffer and Be Still: Women in the Victorian Age*, Bloomington: Indiana University Press.

—— Vicinus, M. (ed.) (1980) *A Widening Sphere: Changing Roles of Victorian Women*, London: Methuen.

Walkowitz, J.R. (1980) *Prostitution and Victorian Society: Women, Class and the State*, Cambridge: Cambridge University Press.

—— (1982) 'Male vice and feminist virtue: feminism and the politics of prostitution in nineteenth century Britain', *History Workshop Journal*, 13, Spring: 79–93.

Watt, I. (1957) *The Rise of the Novel: Studies in Defoe, Richardson and Fielding*, London: Chatto & Windus.

Weeks, J. (1981) *Sex, Politics and Society: The Regulation of Sexuality Since 1800*, London: Longman.

Wilson, A. (1980) 'The infancy of the history of childhood: an appraisal of Philippe Ariès', *History and Theory*, 19: 132–53.

Winn, M. (1977) *The Plug-In Drug*, Harmondsworth: Penguin.

—— (1984) *Children Without Childhood: Growing Up Too Fast in the World of Sex and Drugs*, Harmondsworth: Penguin.

Woodhead, M (1990) 'Psychology and the cultural construction of children's needs' in James, A. and Prout, A. (eds) *Constructing and Reconstructing Childhood: Contemporary Issues in the Sociological Study of Childhood*, London: Falmer Press.

Wordsworth, W. (1936) *The Poetical Works of Wordsworth*, edited by Ernest de Selincourt, London: Oxford University Press.

Wrigley, E.A. and Schofield, R. (1981) *The Population History of England, 1541-1711*, London: Edward Arnold.

Yolton, J.W. (1985) *John Locke: An Introduction*, Oxford: Blackwell.

—— and J.S. (eds) (1989) *Some Thoughts Concerning Education by John Locke*, Oxford: Clarendon Press.

Index

1917
207
128
79